Contents

SECTION VIII: RESTORATIVE AND LABORATORY MATERIALS AND TECHNIQUES

SECTION IX: DENTAL PRACTICE MANAGEMENT

Part 2: Evaluation of Chapter Knowledge Checklists

Instructor's Manual
to Accompany

Dental Assisting:
A Comprehensive Approach

FOURTH EDITION

Donna J. Phinney, CDA, FADAA, BA, MEd

Judy H. Halstead, CDA, BA

DELMAR
CENGAGE Learning

Australia • Brazil • Japan • Korea • Mexico • Singapore • Spain • United Kingdom • United States

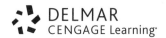

Instructor's Manual to Accompany:
Dental Assisting: A Comprehensive
Approach, Fourth Edition
Donna J. Phinney and Judy H. Halstead

Vice President, Editorial: Dave Garza

Director of Learning Solutions: Matthew Kane

Acquisitions Editor: Tari Broderick

Managing Editor: Marah Bellegarde

Senior Product Manager: Darcy M. Scelsi

Editorial Assistant: Nicole Manikas

Vice President, Marketing: Jennifer Baker

Marketing Manager: Scott Chrysler

Production Director: Wendy Troeger

Production Manager: Andrew Crouth

Senior Content Project Manager:
    Kenneth McGrath

Senior Art Director: Jack Pendleton

Technology Project Manager:
    Brandon Dingeman

Production Technology Analyst:
    Mary Colleen Liburdi

For product information and technology assistance, contact us at
Cengage Learning Customer & Sales Support, 1-800-354-9706

For permission to use material from this text or product,
submit all requests online at **www.cengage.com/permissions**
Further permissions questions can be e-mailed to
permissionrequest@cengage.com

Library of Congress Control Number: 2011943937

ISBN-13: 978-1-1115-43006

ISBN-10: 1-1115-4300-3

Delmar
5 Maxwell Drive
Clifton Park, NY 12065-2919
USA

Cengage Learning is a leading provider of customized learning solutions with office locations around the globe, including Singapore, the United Kingdom, Australia, Mexico, Brazil, and Japan. Locate your local office at:
international.cengage.com/region

Cengage Learning products are represented in Canada by Nelson Education, Ltd.

To learn more about Delmar, visit **www.cengage.com/delmar**

Purchase any of our products at your local college store or at our preferred online store **www.cengagebrain.com**

Notice to the Reader
Publisher does not warrant or guarantee any of the products described herein or perform any independent analysis in connection with any of the product information contained herein. Publisher does not assume, and expressly disclaims, any obligation to obtain and include information other than that provided to it by the manufacturer. The reader is expressly warned to consider and adopt all safety precautions that might be indicated by the activities described herein and to avoid all potential hazards. By following the instructions contained herein, the reader willingly assumes all risks in connection with such instructions. The publisher makes no representations or warranties of any kind, including but not limited to, the warranties of fitness for particular purpose or merchantability, nor are any such representations implied with respect to the material set forth herein, and the publisher takes no responsibility with respect to such material. The publisher shall not be liable for any special, consequential, or exemplary damages resulting, in whole or part, from the readers' use of, or reliance upon, this material.

Printed in the United States of America
1 2 3 4 5 6 7 14 13 12

Message to the Instructor

One of our major roles as educators of dental assistants is to prepare students for Dental Assisting National Board, Inc. (DANB) certification and to be proficient in the skills of their profession upon graduation. To attain that goal, we should facilitate student learning as accurately and efficiently as possible.

This can be achieved through the use of a well-developed and complete learning system that uses various learning media that account for the different ways in which today's students learn. The textbook, *Dental Assisting: A Comprehensive Approach, Fourth Edition*, and supporting and instructional materials are designed as guides to building the attitudes, behavior, and skills necessary for a successful career as a dental assistant. This extensive learning system is designed to build on the instructor's already vast and considerable education and training. The text is complemented with a comprehensive student *Workbook to Accompany Dental Assisting*, *StudyWARE*™ student practice CD, *Interactive Skills and Procedures* student CD, *Dental Assisting Instruments Guide*, *Dental Assisting Materials Guide*, *CourseMate*, *Dental Terminology 3e*, *Dental Assisting Coloring Book*, *Dental Assisting Video Series*, and *Delmar's Dental Assisting Exam Review*. The instructor support materials can be found online and consist of an Instructor's Manual, chapter presentations in Power Point, a computerized test bank, an image library, and handouts and worksheets as well as various tools to aid in use of the book and in lesson planning. With the help of this Instructor's Manual, these components are easily structured into a classroom setting, with the expertise of a qualified instructor.

THE LEARNING SYSTEM

The components of the learning system were developed with today's learner in mind. The authors and Cengage Learning recognize that students learn in different ways—they read, write, listen, watch, interact, and practice. For this reason, we've created a variety of products learners can use to fully comprehend and retain what they're taught. This Instructor's Manual ties the components together, making classroom integration easy and fun.

The Text
This text delivers comprehensive coverage of dental assisting theory and practice, supported by full-color illustrations and photographs throughout and 152 step-by-step procedures in nine sections. Section I—Introduction—introduces learners to the profession, its history, communication, and legal issues. Section II—Prevention and Nutrition—covers general techniques to maintain health and wellness of the oral cavity and the dentition. Section III—Basic Dental Sciences—covers the basics of dental anatomy, embryology, histology, tooth morphology, charting, and microbiology, creating a foundation on which learners can move forward to skills training. Section IV—Preclinical Dental Skills—prepares students in the areas of infection control, hazardous materials management, patient care, pharmacology, and emergency management, critical elements to the profession. Section V—Clinical Dental Procedures—covers chairside assisting, instruments, and the management of pain and anxiety. Section VI—Dental Radiography—provides

updated information on radiographic techniques and procedures, including the latest on digital radiography. Section VII—Dental Specialties—introduces learners to the specialized areas of endodontics, oral and maxillofacial surgery, oral pathology, orthodontics, pediatric dentistry, periodontics, fixed prosthodontics, cosmetic dentistry, and removable prosthodontics. Section VIII—Restorative and Laboratory Materials and Techniques—covers chairside restorative materials and techniques and laboratory and impression materials and techniques. Section IX—Dental Practice Management—contains coverage of dental office management, dental computer software, dental insurance, and legal and ethical considerations, important components for managing a dental practice properly, as well as employment portfolios. Advanced chairside functions such as dam placement, coronal polishing, and retraction cord placement are covered in the individual chapters where that coverage would be provided in states that are teaching expanded functions.

"How to Use this Text" and "How to Use StudyWARE™" sections guide instructors and students through the text and software programs, enabling teaching and learning in the best way possible. Appendices and a comprehensive glossary and index are also included.

Chapters include the following pedagogical features:

- Chapter outline
- Specific Instructional Objectives
- Key terms (key terms also appear in color in the text)
- Pronunciation of difficult terms the first time they appear in the text
- Introduction
- Step-by-step procedures with icons indicating handwashing, gloves, mask and protective eyewear, basic setup, and expanded functions
- In-text icons identifying legal, safety, technology, and global/cultural issues, and DANB exam components
- Boxed information containing tips and summaries
- Summary
- Case studies
- Web activity boxes
- Review questions, including critical thinking

Dental Assisting Interactive Skills and Procedures (Order # 978-1-11154-3037)

A skills CD, purchased separately or optionally available packaged with the text, offers activities that simulate dental assisting skills such as dental charting, tray setup, radiograph mounting, and taking vital signs. These activities give learners a chance to practice and test their understanding of content in the text.

Instructor's Manual (Order # 978-1-1115-43006)

The Instructor's Manual ties the learning system together, providing the traditional components of course objectives, answers to text and workbook questions, skills competency checklist sheets to gauge student achievement, and teaching strategies.

- Instructor Companion Website
  An Instructor Companion Website is available to facilitate classroom preparation, presentation, and testing. This content can be accessed through your Instructor SSO account.
  To set-up your account:

  - Go to www.cengagebrain.com/login
  - Choose **Create a New Faculty Account**.
  - Next you will need to select your **Institution**.
  - Complete your personal **Account Information**.
  - Accept the **License Agreement**.
  - Choose **Register**.
  - Your account will be pending validation—you will receive an e-mail notification when the validation process is complete.
  - If you are unable to find your institution, complete an **Account Request Form**.

Once your account is set up or if you already have an account:

- ▶ Go to www.cengagebrain.com/login.
- ▶ Enter your e-mail address and password and select **Sign In**.
- ▶ Search for your book by author, title, or ISBN.
- ▶ Select the book and click **Continue**.
- ▶ You will receive a list of available resources for the title you selected.
- ▶ Choose the resources you would like and click **Add to My Bookshelf**.

Components available on the Instructor Companion site include a(n):

- ▶ Computerized test bank, a 2,300-question bank with questions geared to text chapters and the DANB exam
- ▶ Instructor presentations on PowerPoint with talking points, designed to support and facilitate classroom instruction
- ▶ Electronic version of the *Instructor's Manual*, so notes and ideas can be customized
- ▶ Electronic image library containing files of hundreds of images from the text
- ▶ Dental assisting curriculum that cross-references all of Cengage Learning's dental assisting materials to create a dynamic learning system
- ▶ Correlation guide to help make a smooth transition from the third edition to the fourth edition
- ▶ Conversion grids to help make the change from one of our competitor's books to our books
- ▶ Additional Handouts on Key Terms Review and additional activities such as crossword puzzles, word searches, and matching and labeling exercises
- ▶ Skill checklists to use for student evaluation.

Student Workbook (Order # 978-1-11154-2993)

The workbook, which corresponds to the text, contains chapter objectives, summaries, exercises in a variety of formats, and skill sheets to test competencies.

Web Tutors

The self-paced Web Tutor modules include chapter objectives, chapter presentations on PowerPoint, quizzes, Web links, critical thinking questions, a discussion board, and video links. Both Web CT (order # 978-1-11154-3044) and Blackboard (order # 978-1-11154-3051) formats are available.

CourseMate

CourseMate complements your textbook with several robust and noteworthy components:

- ▶ An interactive eBook, with highlighting, note taking, and search capabilities
- ▶ Interactive and engaging learning tools including flashcards, quizzes, videos, games, PowerPoint presentations, and much more!
- ▶ Engagement Tracker, a first-of-its-kind tool that monitors student participation and retention in the course.

To access CourseMate content:

- ▶ Go to www.cengagebrain.com
- ▶ For an Internet access code (Order # 978-1-11154-3082)
- ▶ For a Print access code (Order # 978-1-11154-3075)

Other supporting materials include:

- ▶ *Dental Terminology, 3rd Edition* (Charline Dofka) (Order # 978-1-13301-9718)
- ▶ *Dental Assisting Coloring Book* (Donna Phinney and Judy Halstead) (Order # 978-1-4390-5931-9)
- ▶ *Dental Assisting Instrument Guide* (Donna Phinney and Judy Halstead) (Order # 978-1-4180-52003)
- ▶ *Dental Assisting Materials Guide* (Donna Phinney and Judy Halstead) (Order # 978-1-4180-5199-0)
- ▶ *Dental Assisting Video Series* (Order # 978-1-4180-2963-0)

When you use all these components together, you'll discover an innovative, comprehensive system of teaching and learning that prepares students for success in the 21st century.

Each textbook comes with a free *StudyWARE*^{TM} disk, bound in the back. The disk contains over 1,500 exercises, utilizing a variety of formats—multiple choice, short answer, true/false, matching, labeling, and concentration—to further reinforce content. "How to Use This Text" and "How to Use StudyWare™" sections guide instructors and students through the text, enabling teaching and learning in the best way possible.

INSTRUCTOR'S MANUAL ORGANIZATION

The Instructor's Manual has been designed to make it easy for instructors to use the entire learning system. It provides the traditional chapter objectives, answers to case study review questions, answers to text and student workbook questions, and evaluation of chapter knowledge checklists. The lecture outlines correlate to the PowerPoint presentations provided for each chapter, the preparatory content offers suggestions for materials and personnel to utilize to teach the content, and the teaching strategies provide suggestions for in-class activities and assignments to aid in preparing for the presentation of the content. More importantly, it provides a framework for integrating all components of the learning system. As a dental assisting instructor, you will find that the following instructional suggestions and supportive materials facilitate your organizing a well-planned lesson.

OUTCOME- OR COMPETENCY-BASED EDUCATION

For dental assisting instructors, outcome- or competency-based education has become an integral part of dental assisting programs and is used to describe the performance and skill levels a student must possess to be considered competent and at entry level for employment. When students have the opportunity to participate in a program of study that is outcome- or competency-based, they know exactly what is expected of them, making the transition from the classroom to the world of work easier.

Performance will be the primary evidence of achievement, as well as the instrument used to measure student knowledge and competency. The student's education is directed toward preparing him or her to perform prescribed tasks of dental assisting under the conditions of the "real" world and at a level of competency (accuracy and timeliness) necessary to pass the DANB exam and become entry-level dental assistants.

INSTRUCTIONAL IDEAS AND SUGGESTIONS

1. **Levels of Learning:** Each student works at a different level. Learn to recognize these levels and base your presentation on this information. Start at an initial level and continue to build to a higher level. You will enjoy the class more and your students will benefit from this form of teaching.

2. **Visual Aids:** Use all available visual aids (e.g., videos, transparencies, etc.). Cengage Learning has excellent supportive materials such as videos, transparencies, PowerPoint presentations, CourseMate, and an image library that can make a difference to the students when you share with them the practical application of how to do a procedure. These aids are also great for students who learn visually. Remember, many of today's students were brought up in the television and computer age, a visual environment where information is broken up into smaller, appealing pieces. Multimedia instruction also presents material in a variety of formats, ensuring that all students with all learning styles have an opportunity to understand and internalize instruction.

3. **Lecture:** Lecture(s) should be prepared carefully so that you are presenting a thorough and well-organized presentation. The lecture is the most common method of instruction but can be the most boring for students. Be creative in your presentations and involve your students often in the discussion. Also use visual aids in your lectures.

4. **Exams:** Depending on the type of program that has been set up for teaching the dental assisting program, exams may be a part of the instructional material. Exams can be done at the beginning or end of class. The exam should provide the instructor feedback as to whether or not the student understands the material presented.

5. **A. Laboratory Instruction:** This portion of the course is really fun for the instructor. The demonstrations should relate to the sequential steps in any procedure. (Remember to emphasize that procedures

or functions should always be accomplished without trauma to the patient when dealing with soft or hard tissues of the oral cavity.) Encourage the students to ask questions during the demonstration and remember: DON'T ASSUME that they know the information you are teaching. Test students' knowledge of what they've just seen by asking questions throughout and after the procedure. Make sure you're explaining the "whys" behind your actions. Students learn more quickly and retain that knowledge better when they understand the rationale or theory behind their practice.

B. **Student Participation:** After a demonstration has been given, it is time for the students to practice the functions and prepare for the clinical checkoff.

C. **Clinical Checkoff:** Clinical checkoff, or practice, is where the students have the opportunity to perform the procedures they were shown in class (lab). Success in this area means that students will be able to practice these functions in a dental office according to the functions and criteria of the DANB, the individual dental office, and their states.

D. **Evaluation:** Evaluation by the instructor is very valuable to the student. The instructor assesses progress and determines whether students are ready for the next level or the next procedure. Formal evaluation of a procedure can be conducted using checklists that list those functions/procedures needed to complete an area or subject. Instructors can simply "check off" that a step has been completed satisfactorily, or they can assign a measure (for instance, 1–5) indicating students' level of performance. (The measuring system can also be used to assign "weights" to various steps, from less to more to most critical.) Use the Skill Competency Assessment checklists in the *Workbook* (also available on the Instructor Companion Website) to evaluate a student's performance of a specific procedure. Use the Evaluation of Chapter Knowledge checklists found in this manual to review and assess a student's knowledge of the concepts and objectives presented in any given chapter.

6. **Guest Speakers:** Guest speakers can really be a lot of fun and very informative. They provide students with exposure to the profession and its real-life demands. They also offer an opportunity for students to get to know the practitioners in their community—people with whom they may be working.

7. **Field Trips:** Field trips can be another type of informative function for students. Possible field trips could include a trip to an oral surgery office, an orthodontics office, a dental lab, or a dental supply house. The professionals here can really share with the student the goings-on in a dental practice. Learn to be creative. As an instructor you'll also need to do the following:

▶ Arrange the visit with the site and your school's administration.
▶ Have students prepare some questions to ask of the staff members while at the site.
▶ Have students complete a summary of their experience to share with the class.
▶ After the trip, send a thank-you note to the site from the students and yourself.

HEALTH AND SAFETY

Be sure that students are working in a safe environment. Always keep equipment maintained and materials up-to-date. It is the responsibility of the instructor to keep things safe. To maintain safety, you must be aware of current and new regulations regarding the Occupational Safety and Health Act (OSHA), safe and proper handling of laboratory equipment, chairside skills, and proper procedures/objectives regarding radiation safety for the operator and the patient.

If you are not current or sure of new standards relating to the profession of dental assisting, contact OSHA or the American Dental Association (ADA) directly for information, seminars (courses), and any other educational programs available to bring you up-to-date so that you can keep things safe for your students and yourself.

CONCULSION

By using these suggestions, this Instructor's Manual, and the entire learning system, you are ensuring your students' success in your program, on their DANB exam, and in their profession. We wish you and your students our best and would love to hear from you. Good luck!

HOW TO USE STUDYWARE

StudyWare™ is includes learning activities, quizzes, animations, and video clips to help study key concepts from *Dental Assisting: A Comprehensive Approach, Fourth Edition* and to test comprehension.

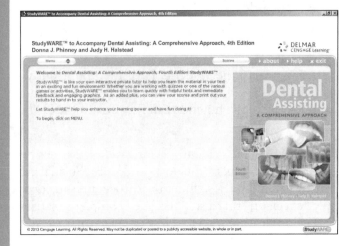

MAIN MENU

The main menu follows the chapter organization of the book—which makes it easy to find your way around. Just click on the button for the chapter you want, and then click on the activity that you wish to practice.

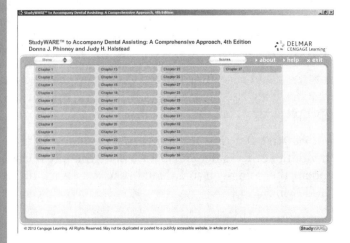

Minimum System Requirements

- Microsoft Windows XP w/SP 2, Windows Vista w/SP 1, Windows 7
- Mac OS X 10.4, 10.5, or 10.6
- Processor: Minimum required by Operating System
- Memory: Minimum required by Operating System
- Hard Drive Space: 410MB
- Screen resolution: 1024 x 768 pixels
- CD-ROM drive
- Sound card & listening device required for audio features
- Flash Player 10. The Adobe Flash Player is free and can be downloaded from http://www.adobe.com/products/flashplayer/

Windows Setup Instructions

1. Insert disc into CD-ROM drive. The software installation should start automatically. If it does not, go to step 2.
2. From My Computer, double-click the icon for the CD drive.
3. Double-click the *setup.exe* file to start the program.

Mac Setup Instructions

1. Insert disc into CD-ROM drive.
2. Once the disc icon appears on your desktop, double click on it to open it.
3. Double-click the *StudyWare*™ to start the program.

Technical Support:
Telephone: 1-800-645-3565
Monday–Thursday 8:30 a.m.–9:00 p.m., Friday 8:30 a.m.–6:00 p.m. (Eastern Time)
Web: www.cengage.com/support

StudyWare™ is a trademark used herein under license.
Microsoft® and Windows® are registered trademarks of the Microsoft Corporation.
Pentium® is a registered trademark of the Intel® Corporation.

EXERCISES AND ACTIVITIES

StudyWare™ acts as a private tutor. For each exercise, it chooses from a bank of over 1,500 questions covering all 37 chapters. Putting these exercises to work for you is simple:

- Choose either the practice or test mode. You'll encounter a series of questions from the chapter. The questions are generated randomly so you can practice more than once and receive different questions each time.
- Question styles include multiple choice, fill-in-the-blank, matching, and true/false.
- Instant feedback in practice mode tells you whether you are right or wrong—and helps you learn quickly by explaining why the answer is correct or incorrect.
- Your test scores are saved and can be reviewed to determine the questions you missed.

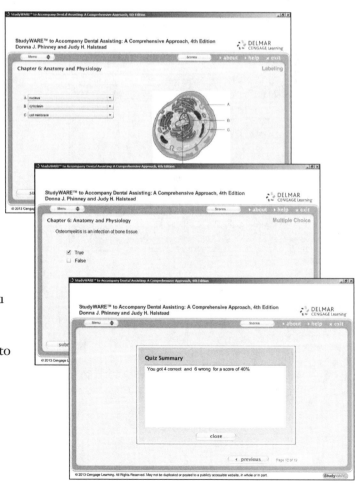

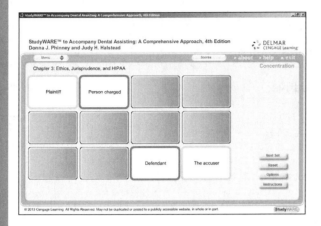

FUN AND GAMES

- Championship Game—A Jeopardy-style quiz game that can be played solo or with a partner.
- Concentration—Match terms and key concepts to their corresponding definitions or descriptions.
- Hangman—Review spelling and vocabulary by choosing the correct letters to spell dental words appropriate to the chapter.
- Media—Review video clips and animations to reinforce comprehension of the concepts discussed within the chapters.

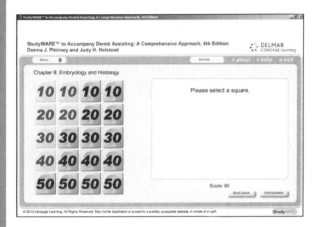

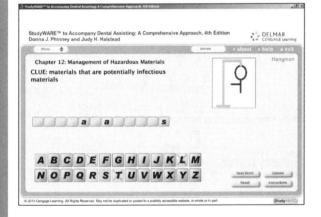

HOW TO USE DENTAL ASSISTING INTERACTIVE SKILLS AND PROCEDURES SOFTWARE

Dental Assisting Interactive Skills and Procedures Software has been designed to help the student practice the essential dental assisting skills covered in *Dental Assisting: A Comprehensive Approach, 4th edition*. In these interactive exercises the student will read patient profiles and then take blood pressures, complete oral and periodontal charts, mount radiographs, and set up dental trays for many different types of procedures, such as amalgam and composite restorations, oral surgery, periodontics, endodontics, and prosthodontics.

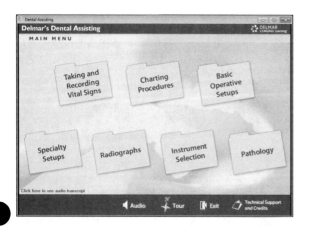

MAIN MENU

From the main menu, you can select the type of skill you want to practice. You can choose Taking and Recording Vital Signs, Charting Procedures, Basic Operative Setups, Specialty Setups, Radiographs, Pathology, or Instrument Identification.

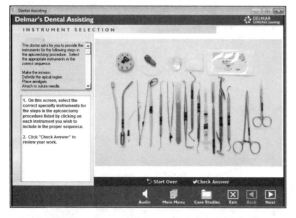

CASE STUDY MENU

Many of the exercises are based on case studies of individual patients. From the case study menu, choose a patient file and then practice the dental assisting skill for that patient's procedure. When you are finished with one case, you can choose another or go back to the main menu.

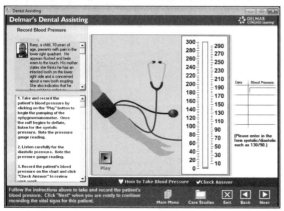

TAKING AND RECORDING VITAL SIGNS

The Vital Signs exercises let you practice taking and recording blood pressure and TPR (temperature, pulse, and respiration). In the simulated blood pressure exercise, you can read the patient's chart, then pump up the sphygmomanometer, watch the pressure gauge, listen for the systolic and diastolic pressure, and record the patient's blood pressure on the chart.

CHARTING PROCEDURES

The Charting Procedures exercises will give you practice filling in interactive oral exam and periodontal charts while listening to the dentist's dictation. You can vary the rate of the dentist's dictation, increasing your skill by beginning with very slow and progressing to normal speed dictation.

BASIC OPERATIVE SETUPS

The Basic Operative Setups exercises will give you practice assembling anesthetic syringes, punching and assembling dental dams, and setting up dental trays for amalgam and composite restorations. In the anesthetic exercises, you will choose the correct anesthetic carpules, the correct syringe, and the correctly assembled syringe for the patient. The dental dam exercises ask you to select the correct armamentarium for the tray, correctly punch the dental dam, and choose the properly assembled dental dam for the patient.

SPECIALTY SETUPS

The Specialty Setups exercises will give you practice in recognizing the appropriate tray setups for the specific procedures the patients are going to have done. You can review many different trays set up for oral surgery, periodontics, endodontics, orthodontics, and prosthodontics, and then choose the correct tray for the patient's procedure.

RADIOGRAPHS

The Radiographs exercises will give you practice in mounting radiographs. In each Mounting Radiographs exercise, you are given a full set of x-rays and you identify them, rotate and position them, and place them correctly in the mount.

PATHOLOGY IDENTIFICATION

This exercise presents you with a series of images and you must choose the correct name of the disease/disorder represented. This will help you to learn the various pathologies that may be encountered in the dental field. It is important for the dental assistant to be alert to abnormal conditions and to update the patient's history and communicate any concerns to the dentist.

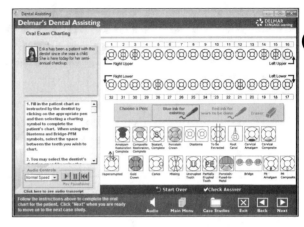

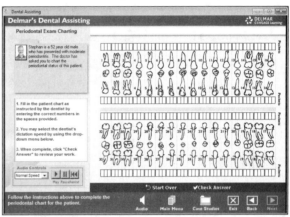

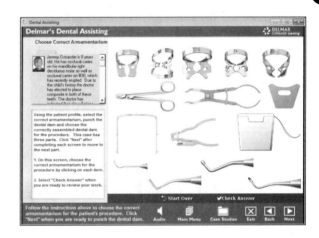

Minimum System Requirements for Skills and Procedures Software:

- ▶ Intel Pentium processor (or compatible) 500 MHz
- ▶ Supported Operating Systems
  - –Windows XP SP2 or higher
  - –Windows Vista
  - –Windows 7
- ▶ RAM: 256 MB or more recommended
- ▶ 275 MB or more free hard disk space
- ▶ CD-ROM or DVD drive

Graphics card that is capable of displaying 800 x 600 pixels resolution with 16-bit color or greater

Set-up Instructions for Skills and Procedures Software:
Insert the *Dental Assisting Interactive Skills and Procedures* CD-ROM.
Double-Click on your My Computer icon on the desktop, then double-click on the CD-ROM drive icon.
Double-click on the setup.exe file to start the installation. Follow the prompts from there.

Preparatory and Lesson Planning

Introduction to the Dental Profession

SPECIFIC INSTRUCTIONAL OBJECTIVES

1. Review dental disease and dentistry from the "beginning of time."

2. Identify the items on the timeline of dental history.

3. Name the individuals who had a great impact on the profession of dentistry.

4. Identify the people who promoted education and organized dentistry.

5. Explain what DDS and DMD stand for.

6. Identify the nine specialties of dentistry.

7. Describe, generally, the career skills performed by dental assistants, dental hygienists, and dental laboratory technicians.

8. List the education required for, and the professional organizations that represent, each dental career path.

PREPARATORY

Personnel

Primary instructor who is knowledgeable about the history of dental assisting and understands the information dental assistants need to know to care for dental patients.

Suggested Audiovisual and Resource Materials

DVDs or videos on the history of dental assisting or dentistry.

▶ *Workbook:* Chapter 1.

▶ *Image Library:* Provides images from Chapter 1 of the textbook that can be used via computer, integrated into PowerPoint presentations, or as transparencies to provide visual support for classroom instruction.

▶ *Computerized Test Bank:* Provides test questions for Chapter 1 and related material on the Dental Assisting National Board (DANB) examination.

▶ *CourseMate:* Additional practice exercises, as well as games, that further reinforce Chapter 1 content can be found on the CourseMate Web site.

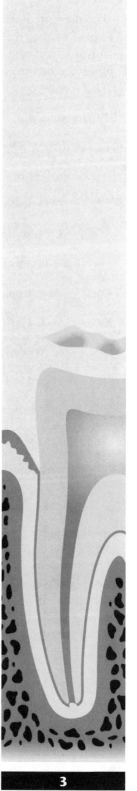

❯ *Dental Terminology, Third Edition:* Chapter 1, Introduction to Dental Terminology, and Chapter 4, Practice and Facility Setups.

❯ *Recommended minimum time to complete Chapter 1:* 3 to 4 hours, depending on depth of information the instructor wishes to provide.

LECTURE OUTLINE CORRELATED TO INSTRUCTOR PRESENTATIONS IN POWERPOINT

The presentations provided contain lecture notes. The notes can be viewed in PowerPoint when viewing the slides in either the normal or outline view. To print the slides with the notes: From your print box look for the "Print What" and change the drop-down to "Notes Pages." A new feature called "Dental Checks" has been interspersed throughout the presentations to keep the student engaged in the materials during the lecture. This feature contains a quick question followed by the answer to stimulate a brief discussion.

1. Introduction to the Dental Profession

2. History of Dentistry—discuss early developments significant to dentistry (Slide 2)

    a. Early times

        i. Herodotus

        ii. Hesi-Re

        iii. Hippocrates

            1. Book *On Affections*

            2. Oath of Hippocrates

        iv. Aristotle

            1. Oral hygiene

    b. Later Progress of Dentistry—discuss further developments of significance in later years (Slides 3 and 4)

        i. Guy de Chauliac

            1. Surgeon from France

            2. Rules for oral hygiene

        ii. Leonardo da Vinci

            1. First to distinguish between molars and premolars

        iii. Pierre Fauchard

            1. Founder of modern dentistry

            2. Rejected idea of tooth worm

            3. Treated caries and diseased gingiva

        iv. Wilhelm Conrad Roentgen

            1. Discovered x-rays

3. Progress of Dentistry in the United States—discuss the key events that shaped dentistry in the United States (Slides 6 through 8)

   a. Robert Woofendale and John Baker

      i. First to advertise dental services

   b. John Greenwood

      i. George Washington's favorite dentist

      ii. Made George Washington's dental prosthesis

   c. Paul Revere

      i. Created artificial teeth and surgical instruments

   d. Josiah Flagg

      i. Skilled surgeon

      ii. Constructed the dental chair

   e. James B. Morrison

      i. Created first dental engine with handpiece, motor, and foot treadle

4. Education and Organized Dentistry—discuss the key events that shaped educational requirements in the dental professions (Slides 9 through 12)

   a. Horace H. Hayden

      i. Writer and lecturer on dental topics

   b. Chapin A. Harris

      i. Created and contributed to library of dental literature

   c. Dr. Greene Vardiman Black

      i. "Grand old man of dentistry"

      ii. Invented machines and instruments used in dentistry

   d. Lucy Beaman Hobbs

   e. Dr. Robert Tanner Freeman

   f. Ida Gray

   g. George Franklin Grant

   h. American Dental Association (ADA)

      i. Horace Hayden and Chapin Harris organized this nationwide association of dentists

      ii. *American Journal of Dental Science*

      iii. Today, each state has a local or regional ADA branch office

5. The Dental Team—discuss the educational requirements and role of each dental team member

   a. Dentists (Slides 14 through 25)

      i. Requirements

         1. Undergraduate education

         2. Graduation from a dental school approved by the ADA, Commission on Dental Accreditation

      ii. Education

         1. 3 to 4 years of undergraduate work

         2. 4 years of dental school

            a. 5 years required at Harvard University

      iii. Dental Specialties

         1. Dental public health

            a. Specialty concerned with the prevention of dental disease

            b. Public health dentist works with the community to promote dental health

         2. Endodontics

            a. Specialty concerned with the pathology and morphology of the dental pulp and surrounding tissues due to injury and disease

         3. Oral and maxillofacial pathology

            a. Specialty concerned with the diagnosis and nature of the diseases that affect the oral cavity

         4. Oral and maxillofacial radiology

            a. Images and data produced by all modalities of radiant energy

               i. For diagnosing and management of disorders of the oral and maxillofacial region

         5. Oral and maxillofacial surgery

            a. Specialty concerned with the diagnosis and surgical treatment of the oral and maxillofacial region due to injury, disease, and defects

         6. Orthodontics and dentofacial orthopedics

            a. Specialty concerned with the diagnosis, supervision, guidance, and correction of malocclusion in the dentofacial structures

         7. Pediatric dentistry

            a. Specialty concerned with the prevention of oral disease and the diagnosis and treatment of oral disease in children

               i. From birth through adolescence

8. Periodontics

    a. Specialty concerned with the diagnosis and treatment of the diseases of the supporting and surrounding tissues of the tooth

9. Prosthodontics

    a. Specialty concerned with the diagnosis, restoration, and maintenance of oral functions

b. Dental Assistants (Slides 27 through 29)

    i. Dr. C. Edmund Kells

        1. Hired a "Lady Assistant" to be "quick, quiet, gentle, and attentive"

        2. "Ladies in Attendance"

    ii. Dental Assisting National Board (DANB)

    iii. Certified Dental Assistant (CDA)

    iv. Dental receptionists

    v. American Dental Assistants Association (ADAA)

    vi. Juliette Southard

        1. Founder and first president of the American Dental Assistants Association

c. Dental Hygienists (Slide 30)

    i. Dr. Alfred Civilon Fones

        1. Developed first school of dental hygiene in 1913

    ii. American Dental Hygienists' Association (ADHA)

d. Dental Laboratory Technicians (Slides 31 and 32)

    i. Many are graduates of a 2-year ADA-accredited dental laboratory technician program

    ii. Formal education is not required

    iii. Examination to become certified dental technicians (CDTs)

    iv. American Dental Laboratory Technician Association (ADLTA)

e. Other Members of the Dental Team (Slide 33)

    i. Dental service technicians

    ii. Dental representatives

    iii. Dental supply companies and representatives

TEACHING STRATEGIES

1. Consider providing photos of the individuals who have impacted the field of dentistry and who are discussed in this chapter. Photos can be found in the image library. These photos can be incorporated into the PowerPoint presentations. A PowerPoint slide showing just the images of historians in the dental field can be presented in class as a pop quiz.

CASE STUDY ANSWERS

1. Beginning in 1885, female dental assistants were accepted into the profession. Before then, dental assistants were primarily male.

2. Dental assistants went from being "ladies in attendance," where they primarily offered support and comfort to the patient, to today's dental assistants, who assist the dentist in chairside procedures and perform invasive procedures, such as placing retraction cords and dental dams.

3. Dental assistants can obtain a national credential from the Dental Assisting National Board. Credentials include certified dental assistant (CDA), certified preventive assistant (CDPA) and certified orthodontic assistant (COA). In some states, registration credentials are available. In these states, an assistant can become a registered dental assistant (RDA) or a registered expanded functions dental assistant (REFDA) also known as a registered dental assistant in expanded functions (RDAEF).

TEXTBOOK REVIEW ANSWERS

Multiple Choice

1. d   2. b   3. c   4. a   5. c   6. a   7. c   8. a

9. b   10. a

Critical Thinking

1. Oral and maxillofacial surgeon, endodontist, and prosthodontist.

2. Any of the national dental or dental assistant organizations (see Appendix A for contact information) may be contacted regarding local chapters.

3. Dental hygienist.

CHAPTER 2

Psychology, Communication, and Multicultural Interaction

SPECIFIC INSTRUCTIONAL OBJECTIVES

1. Define psychology and paradigm.

2. Describe the components of the communication process.

3. Describe how the baby boomer generation may differ from generations "X" and "Y."

4. List the skills used in listening.

5. Differentiate the terms used in verbal and nonverbal communication.

6. Demonstrate how the following body language is used in nonverbal communication: spatial, posture, facial expression, gestures, and perception.

7. Discuss how Maslow's hierarchy of needs is used and how it relates to communication in today's dental office.

8. Discuss how defense mechanisms can inhibit communication.

9. Describe some general behaviors of multicultural patient populations.

PREPARATORY

Personnel

Primary instructor who is knowledgeable about psychology, communication, and multicultural interactions, and understands the information the dental assistant needs to know when caring for and interacting with dental patients and other dental team members.

Suggested Audiovisual and Resource Materials

DVDs or videos demonstrating skills such as communicating with patients and coworkers, verbal versus nonverbal communication, body language, and behaviors exhibited by various cultures.

▶ *Workbook:* Chapter 2.

▶ *Image Library:* Provides illustrations from Chapter 2 of the textbook that can be used via computer to provide visual support for the classroom instruction.

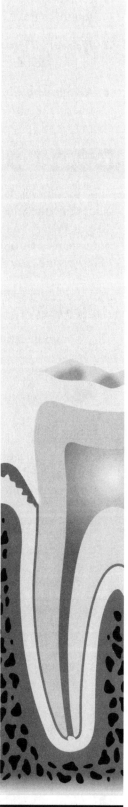

9

▶ *Computerized Test Bank:* Provides test questions for Chapter 2 and related material on the Dental Assisting National Board (DANB) examination.

▶ *StudyWare:* Provides additional review questions and activities for Chapter 2 content that can be found on the companion software disk.

▶ *CourseMate:* Additional practice exercises, as well as games, that further reinforce Chapter 2 content can be found on the CourseMate Web site.

▶ *Delmar's Dental Assisting Exam Review:* Provides additional review material, test questions, and rationales to provide practice for the DANB examination.

▶ *Recommended minimum time to complete Chapter 2:* 3 to 4 hours, depending on depth of information the instructor wishes to provide.

LECTURE OUTLINE CORRELATED TO INSTRUCTOR PRESENTATIONS IN POWERPOINT

The presentations provided contain lecture notes. The notes can be viewed in PowerPoint when viewing the slides in either the normal or outline view. To print the slides with the notes: From your print box look for the "Print What" and change the drop-down to "Notes Pages." A new feature called "Dental Checks" has been interspersed throughout the presentations to keep the student engaged in the materials during the lecture. This feature contains a quick question followed by the answer to stimulate a brief discussion.

1. Psychology and Understanding Individual Paradigms—define and explain psychology and paradigms (Slide 2)

2. Communication (Slide 3)

    a. Verbal

    b. Nonverbal

    c. Listening

3. Communication Process—explain the sender, message, channel, receiver, and feedback concepts, providing examples of each. Have two students demonstrate an interaction and have the class determine whether the communication cycle occurred and whether communication was effective. (Slides 4 and 5)

    i. Sender

    ii. Message

    iii. Channel

    iv. Receiver

    v. Feedback

4. Listening Skills—discuss the various barriers to communication—have students role-play to demonstrate various barriers that may be encountered (Slide 6)

    a. Telephone Listening—play answering machine messages and have students write down what they hear (Slide 7)

5. Understanding Different Generations (Slide 8)

    a. Baby Boomers

    b. Generation "X"

    c. Generation "Y"

6. Verbal and Nonverbal Communication—explain and provide examples of the various nonverbal clues people will exhibit when communicating. Have students role-play these situations. (Slide 9)

    i. Territoriality or Spatial Relation

    ii. Posture and Position

    iii. Facial Expression

    iv. Gestures

    v. Perception

7. Maslow's Hierarchy of Needs—discuss each of the levels of the hierarchy. Provide examples for each. Create a PowerPoint presentation that provides a scenario and have students determine what level of the hierarchy it exemplifies. (Slides 11 through 13)

    i. Survival or Physiological Needs

    ii. Safety Needs

    iii. Belongingness and Love Needs

    iv. Prestige and Esteem Needs

    v. Self-Actualization

8. Defense Mechanisms—discuss the various defense mechanisms that can block effective communication. Have students role-play scenarios where these mechanisms are exhibited. (Slide 14)

9. Culture, Ethnicity, and Race—explain the differences among the terms (Slide 16)

10. Multicultural Interaction—provide examples of typical behaviors customary to a particular group of people and discuss ways to accommodate the behaviors to foster effective communication (Slide 17)

TEACHING STRATEGIES

1. The students can be organized into groups, with each group being responsible for preparing and delivering a presentation on people of a specific culture. Presentations can cover beliefs, behavior, attitudes, customs, languages, symbols, ceremonies, rituals, knowledge, and practices that are distinctive to the particular grouping. The students can present information about the geographical area, economy, and dentistry specifics, including the use of audiovisual aids such as PowerPoint text and images.

2. A quiz or a game such as the word search on the CourseMate or a Web assignment can be required of the students to again review the material and broaden their knowledge base.

CASE STUDY ANSWERS

1. The levels of Maslow's hierarchy of needs that are addressed in this scenario are the lower three levels. The survival or physiological needs as well as the safety needs are due to her home being lost. The belongingness and love needs level is due to her husband leaving.

2. There is always discussion on this topic, but many do feel that the basic levels need to be met before seeking a higher level. In this case study there are several aspects involving different levels. The first area that would need to be addressed would be to find a home and have a place to live.

3. The level in the hierarchy of needs in which the dental office teamwork belongs is the third level, belongingness and love needs.

TEXTBOOK REVIEW ANSWERS

Multiple Choice

1. c   2. d   3. d   4. c   5. b   6. b   7. c   8. c

9. d   10. b

Critical Thinking

1. Defense mechanisms may be denial, regression, and rationalization for justification. To overcome the defense mechanisms, the root reason for the defensive behavior needs to be identified. Once the reason for the defensive behavior is identified it can be addressed in a manner that engages the individual and educates the individual about how to move forward. Individual answers may vary related to how individual students may have responded to this behavior in their own experiences.

2. Some nonverbal forms of communication that may be observed in the dental office include the patient tightening his or her hands on the arms of the chair, a look that may indicate a need the patient has, the patient's posture in the chair, or a muffled noise the patient makes. The intent may be to let the dental assistant know that the patient may need something or is uncomfortable with the treatment.

3. Self-actualization is the highest level on Maslow's hierarchy of needs. At this level individuals seek to be the best they can be. These individuals show spontaneity in their ideas and actions, they are creative, interested in solving problems, appreciate life, harbor no prejudices, and embrace the facts and realities of the world.

4. Refer to Figure 2-8 in the textbook.

Ethics, Jurisprudence, and the Health Information Portability and Accountability Act

SPECIFIC INSTRUCTIONAL OBJECTIVES

1. Identify the difference between civil and criminal law.

2. Define the Dental Practice Act and what it covers.

3. Identify who oversees the Dental Practice Act and how licenses in the dental field are obtained.

4. Define expanded functions.

5. Identify the components of a contract.

6. Identify due care and give examples of malpractice and torts.

7. Define fraud and where it may be seen in the dental office.

8. Identify care that can be given under the Good Samaritan Law.

9. Identify the four areas of the Americans with Disabilities Act.

10. Identify the responsibilities of the dental team in regard to dental records, implied and informed consent, subpoenas, and the statute of limitations.

11. Define ethics and give examples of the American Dental Association and American Dental Assistants Association's principles of ethics.

12. State how dentistry follows ethical principles regarding advertising, professional fees and charges, and professional responsibilities and rights.

13. State how the HIPAA law has impacted the dental office and identify the parameters of the law.

14. Identify how patient health information can be used and disclosed, as well as the rights of the patients.

15. Gain an understanding of the training that the staff must follow to be compliant with the HIPAA laws.

16. Identify the CDT transactions and code sets.

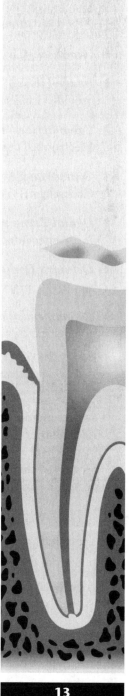

13

Personnel

Primary instructor who is knowledgeable about ethics, jurisprudence, and HIPAA, and understands the information that the dental assistant needs to know when caring for dental patients. The instructor must routinely update the information to be shared with the students on HIPAA.

Suggested Audiovisual and Resource Materials

A number of videos are available that address ethics. Many school video libraries have short videos on this topic. The American Dental Association (ADA) is an excellent resource for updated information on HIPAA and the CDT codes. The ADA publishes the HIPAA Privacy Kit and the updated versions of the CDT codes. Instructors and dental team members can purchase these from the ADA. Information on the most current HIPAA regulations is available on an ongoing basis via the Internet and direct from the government.

▶ *Workbook:* Chapter 3.

▶ *Image Library:* Provides illustrations from Chapter 3 of the textbook that can be used via computer to provide visual support for the classroom instruction.

▶ *Computerized Test Bank:* Provides additional test questions for Chapter 3 content that can be found on the Electronic Classroom Manager.

▶ *CourseMate:* Additional review questions and activities for Chapter 3 content that can be found on the CourseMate Web site.

▶ *Dental Terminology, Third Edition:* Review the last portion of Chapter 20 related to legal and ethics terms for further information and review of concepts presented in the chapter.

▶ *Delmar's Dental Assisting Exam Review:* Provides additional review material, test questions, and rationale to provide practice for the Dental Assisting National Board (DANB) examination.

▶ *Recommended minimum time to complete Chapter 3:* 4 to 5 hours, depending on depth of information that the instructor wishes to cover.

LECTURE OUTLINE CORRELATED TO INSTRUCTOR PRESENTATIONS IN POWERPOINT

The presentations provided contain lecture notes. The notes can be viewed in PowerPoint when viewing the slides in either the normal or outline view. To print the slides with the notes: From your print box look for the "Print What" and change the drop-down to "Notes Pages." A new feature called "Dental Checks" has been interspersed throughout the presentations to keep the student engaged in the materials during the lecture. This feature contains a quick question followed by the answer to stimulate a brief discussion.

1. The Law (Slides 2 through 5)

   a. Civil and Criminal Law—discuss the difference in these two types of law and present examples of each from the field of dentistry

   b. Dental Practice Act—discuss the importance of the act and the specifics of how it relates to the dental assistant

   c. State Board of Dentistry—define the role of the board and the impact of the field of dental assisting; explain licensure and expanded functions

2. The Dentist, the Dental Assistant, and the Law (Slides 7 and 8)

    a. Contracts—discuss the different types of contracts and provide examples of each related to the dental field

    b. Explain what constitutes a termination of a contract

3. Standard of Care (Slides 9 through 14)

    a. Malpractice—define and give an example from dental practice

    b. Torts—define and give an example from dental practice

    c. Assault and Battery—define and give an example from dental practice

    d. Defamation of Character—define and give an example from dental practice

    e. Invasion of Privacy—define and give an example from dental practice

    f. Fraud—define and give an example from dental practice

    g. Good Samaritan Law—define and give an example from dental practice

    h. Child Abuse and Neglect—define and give an example from dental practice

    i. Americans with Disabilities Act—explain the impact of the field of dentistry

4. Dental Records (Slides 16 and 17)

    a. Informed Consent—define and give an example from dental practice

    b. Implied Consent—define and give an example from dental practice

    c. Subpoenas—define

    d. Statute of Limitations—define

5. Ethics (Slides 18 and 19)

    a. Advertising—explain the impact and provide ethical and unethical examples

    b. Professional Fees and Charges—explain and provide examples

    c. Professional Responsibilities and Rights—outline

6. HIPAA (Slides 18 through 39)

    a. The Law—present an overview of the law and the impact on the dental assistant

    b. Transactions and Code Sets (Slide 22)—explain and define

    c. What Does HIPAA Encompass?

    d. Who Must Comply with HIPAA?

    e. Protected Health Information (Slides 26 through 32)

    f. Security Rule (Slide 33)

    g. Office Manual (Slides 34 and 35)

    h. Staff Training and Review

    i. Enforcement of HIPAA (Slides 36 through 39)

    j. Federal Civil and Criminal Penalties for Violations of Patient's Right to Privacy

    k. HIPAA Challenge

7. The American Dental Assistants Association Principles of Ethics and Professional Conduct (Slide 41)

    a. Dental Assistants Following Ethics and Jurisprudence

TEACHING STRATEGIES

1. Chapter contents are presented in the PowerPoint slides, which are found in the Instructor Resource CD. The students will need to have a strong background in HIPAA when they work in the dental offices.

2. A video on ethics can be shown to break up the lecture with PowerPoint information. When covering ethics, have several questions to ask the students and discuss how they should be handled. Two difficult examples follow:

    ∗ Your friend is getting married next summer. His/her soon-to-be spouse had an appointment in your office and disclosed that he or she was HIV positive. Assuming that your friend did not know, what would you do?

    ∗ If the doctor was getting sued over dental treatment performed, and he or she asked you to write something on the chart that you could not remember occurring, would you do that?

Discussion on these topics will bring up a number of other questions, and the instructor can sort through these and get back to what would be ethical and legal to do in these situations.

3. A quiz or a Web assignment can be required of the students to again review the material and broaden their knowledge base.

CASE STUDY ANSWERS

1. Desiree should not discuss this with her best friend due to patient confidentiality.

2. She cannot discuss this with her friend legally.

3. She can discuss this further with her friends boyfriend in the office to share agencies that offer HIV/AIDS education for couples. Most states require a blood test prior to marriage license. The dentist most likely will see this when reviewing the health history. If missed by the dentist, she should bring it to their attention, for the patients' health and to provide the best treatment available. The dentist may have other sources of help for the patient to further investigate.

TEXTBOOK REVIEW ANSWERS

Multiple Choice

1. c   2. b   3. c   4. c   5. a   6. d   7. b   8. a   9. d   10. b

Critical Thinking

1. The standard of care as it applies to dental assistants is to treat all patients with due care or what any reasonable and prudent dental assistant professional in the same circumstances would do. Therefore, if a dental assistant is working on a patient who is in need of additional immediate treatment to the area that is already numb, and the assistant knows that another patient is ready, prudence dictates that the assistant would first complete the immediate necessary treatment.

2. The Good Samaritan Law is for individuals who do not seek payment but render medical assistance to the injured. Dental assistants should have emergency training and be ready and able to provide CPR in an emergency situation. In the context of an emergency, the dental assistant can provide care knowing that this law will protect him or her while providing emergency care.

3. Ethics is the moral law and jurisprudence is the legal law.

4. The HIPAA law is not designed to inhibit patients from signing in for treatment.

5. The practice of using the patient's name when calling her or him back for treatment does not violate HIPAA guidelines.

CHAPTER 4

Oral Health and Preventive Techniques

SPECIFIC INSTRUCTIONAL OBJECTIVES

1. Describe how plaque forms and affects the tooth.

2. Identify oral hygiene tips that will aid each age group.

3. Identify oral hygiene aids, including manual and automatic, available to all patients.

4. Demonstrate the six toothbrushing techniques.

5. Identify types of dental floss and demonstrate flossing technique.

6. Describe fluoride and its use in dentistry.

7. Define fluoridation and describe its effect on tooth development and the posteruption stage.

8. List and explain the forms of fluoride. Describe how to prepare a patient and demonstrate a fluoride application.

PREPARATORY

Personnel

Primary instructor who is knowledgeable about dental disease/caries prevention and available products, and understands the information the dental assistant needs to know when caring for dental patients.

Suggested Audiovisual and Resource Materials

A number of videos are available that cover prevention. The American Dental Association (ADA) is an excellent resource for information on prevention for individuals of all ages. Many videos are available for classroom use, as well as printed materials to accompany the videos. Instructors and dental team members can purchase these from the ADA. You can also find information on the Web and from many suppliers of prevention aids. Some of these companies provide free samples to schools. Many have projects that they have developed for children and adults that aid in learning about oral hygiene.

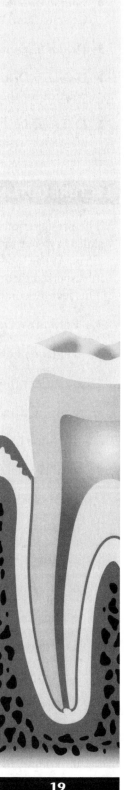

▶ *Workbook:* Chapter 4.

▶ *Image Library:* Provides illustrations from Chapter 4 of the textbook that can be used via computer or as transparencies to provide visual support for classroom instruction.

▶ *Computerized Test Bank:* Provides additional test questions for Chapter 4 and related material on the DANB examination.

▶ *CourseMate:* Additional practice exercises that further reinforce Chapter 4 content can be found on the CourseMate Web site.

▶ *Dental Terminology, Third Edition:* Chapter 7, Examination and Prevention.

▶ *Delmar's Dental Assisting Exam Review:* Additional review material, test questions, and rationales provide practice for the DANB examination.

▶ *Recommended minimum time to complete Chapter 4:* 3 to 4 hours, depending on depth of information the instructor wishes to cover.

LECTURE OUTLINE CORRELATED TO INSTRUCTOR PRESENTATIONS IN POWERPOINT

The presentations provided contain lecture notes. The notes can be viewed in PowerPoint when viewing the slides in either the normal or outline view. To print the slides with the notes: From your print box look for the "Print What" and change the drop-down to "Notes Pages." A new feature called "Dental Checks" has been interspersed throughout the presentations to keep the student engaged in the materials during the lecture. This feature contains a quick question followed by the answer to stimulate a brief discussion.

1. Preventive Dentistry

    a. Plaque Formation (Slide 2)

    b. Patient Motivation (Slide 3)

    c. Age Characteristics (Slides 4 through 11)

    d. Home Care (Slide 13)

2. Oral Hygiene Aids (Slides 14 and 15)

    a. Disclosing Agents

    b. Dentifrice

    c. Mouth Rinses

    d. Chewing Gum

    e. Interdental Aids

3. Toothbrushes and Techniques (Slide 17)

    a. Manual Toothbrushes

    b. Mechanical Toothbrushes

    c. Brushing Techniques for the Manual Toothbrush (Slides 18 through 23)

    d. Tongue Brushing

4. Dental Flossing (Slides 24 and 25)

   a. Types of Floss

   b. Hygienic Care of Prosthetic Devices

5. Oral Hygiene for Patients with Special Needs (Slides 26 and 27)

   a. Pregnant Patients

   b. Patients with Cancer

   c. Patients with Heart Disease

   d. Older Patients

6. Additional Preventive Procedures Performed in the Dental Office

7. Fluoride (Slides 28 through 31)

   a. History of Fluoride in Dentistry

   b. Fluoridation

   c. Effects of Fluoride

   d. Tooth Development

   e. Fluoride in Dental Plaque

   f. Fluoride Toxicity

   g. Benefits of Fluoride

   h. Forms of Fluoride

   i. Topical Fluoride

   j. Advantages and Disadvantages of Fluoride Preparations

   k. Fluoride Rinses

TEACHING STRATEGIES

1. Chapter contents are presented in the PowerPoint slides, which are found in the online Instructor Resources.

2. Videos on prevention can be shown to break up the lecture with PowerPoint information.

3. A quiz or a Web assignment can be required of the students to again review the material and broaden their knowledge base.

4. Have each student take five types of preventive agents (e.g., toothbrushes, flosses, mouth rinses, etc.) and evaluate them according to price, function, ease of use, color, or any other method of evaluation and graph the differences. Students can then write a one-page paper about their findings. Discussion in class after this exercise is typically productive. This exercise requires students to check on such items in local drugstores and supermarkets, an activity that they will continue through their careers to keep current on new items that patients will be exposed to.

CASE STUDY ANSWER

Due to the lack of decay and discoloration of the teeth, a history of fluoride exposure should be evaluated, as was noted in Questions 1 through 5. Asking the case study review questions will aid in diagnosis and treatment.

TEXTBOOK REVIEW ANSWERS

Multiple Choice

1. c	2. d	3. a	4. c	5. d	6. c	7. b	8. a
9. b	10. d						

Critical Thinking

1. The hard candy, because of the exposure time of the teeth to the sugar.

2. No, because fluorosis resulting from overexposure to fluoride occurs during tooth development.

3. The technique used is not important. What counts is that not a single surface of a single tooth is left with plaque on it.

CHAPTER 5

Nutrition

SPECIFIC INSTRUCTIONAL OBJECTIVES

1. Describe how an understanding of nutrition is used in the profession of dental assisting.

2. Define nutrients found in foods, including carbohydrates, fiber, fats, proteins, and amino acids. Explain how they affect oral hygiene.

3. Describe the calorie and the basal metabolic rate.

4. Identify and explain how vitamins, major minerals, and water function in the body.

5. Explain how to interpret food labeling.

6. Discuss the implications of eating disorders.

7. Identify the food sources, functions, and implications of deficiencies of fat-soluble vitamins, water-soluble vitamins, and the seven major minerals.

PREPARATORY

Personnel

Primary instructor who is knowledgeable about dental prevention and nutrition. The instructor should be well informed on eating disorders and food product labeling.

Suggested Audiovisual and Resource Materials

A number of videos are available on nutrition. The American Dietetic Association is an excellent resource for the information on nutrition for people of all ages, including videos for use in classrooms and print materials to accompany the videos. Videos on eating disorders may be available from university and public libraries in the area. Information is also available on the Web. Dietitians will sometimes be available as guest speakers on the topic of nutrition.

▶ *Workbook:* Chapter 5.

▶ *Image Library:* Provides illustrations from Chapter 5 of the textbook that can be used via computer to provide visual support for classroom instruction.

▶ *Computerized Test Bank:* Provides additional test questions for Chapter 5 content that can be found on the companion software disk.

▶ *Delmar's Dental Assisting Exam Review:* Additional review material, test questions, and rationales provide practice for the Dental Assisting National Board (DANB) examination.

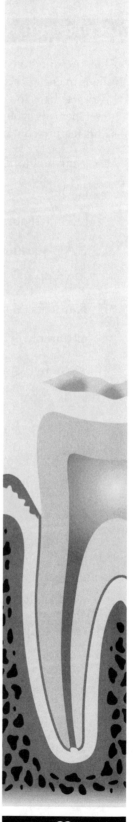

▶ *CourseMate:* Additional practice exercises that further reinforce Chapter 5 content can be found on the CourseMate Web site.

▶ *Recommended minimum time to complete Chapter 5:* 4 to 5 hours, depending on depth of information the instructor wishes to provide.

LECTURE OUTLINE CORRELATED TO INSTRUCTOR PRESENTATIONS IN POWERPOINT

The presentations provided contain lecture notes. The notes can be viewed in PowerPoint when viewing the slides in either the normal or outline view. To print the slides with the notes: From your print box look for the "Print What" and change the drop-down to "Notes Pages." A new feature called "Dental Checks" has been interspersed throughout the presentations to keep the student engaged in the materials during the lecture. This feature contains a quick question followed by the answer to stimulate a brief discussion.

1. Nutrition (Slides 1 and 2)

    a. Diet

    b. Undernourished

    c. Malnutrition

    d. MyPlate

2. Nutrients (Slides 4 through 14)

    a. Carbohydrates

       i. Cariogenic

       ii. Fiber

    b. Fats and Lipids

    c. Proteins

       i. Amino Acids

    d. Vitamins

       i. Fat-soluble

       ii. Water-soluble

    e. Minerals

       i. Major

       ii. Trace

    f. Water

3. Balancing Energy (Slide 14)

    a. Calories

    b. Basal metabolic rate

4. Nutrition Labels (Slide 15)

    a. Serving size

    b. Ingredients

    c. Calories

    d. Fat and cholesterol

    e. Sodium

    f. Carbohydrates

5. Eating Disorders (Slides 16 through 21)

    a. Chronic Dieting Syndrome

    b. Bulimia

    c. Anorexia Nervosa

6. Diet and Culture (Slide 23)

TEACHING STRATEGIES

1. Chapter contents are presented in the PowerPoint slides, which are found in the Instructor Resources to Accompany *Dental Assisting*.

2. Videos on nutrition can be shown to break up the PowerPoint/lecture information. Videos can be obtained from school libraries, the Dairy Council, and many other sources.

3. A quiz or a Web assignment can be required of the students to again review the material and broaden their knowledge base.

4. Place the students in groups and have them develop a presentation on a specific food item (e.g., yogurt, potato chips, orange juice). They can bring samples for the other students to taste, and for comparing brands for calories, trans fat, vitamins, or other pertinent information. A common discovery is that advertised "low-fat" foods are actually higher in fat than other foods typically consumed as snacks, for breakfast, and so on.

5. The students can access ChooseMyPlate.gov online, complete their personal food plan, and evaluate what steps they need to take to become healthier.

CASE STUDY ANSWERS

1. The dental assistant should speak with the dentist in private to share the information he or she learned about Maci.

2. The dentist may believe that the diagnosis of bulimia is accurate based on symptoms.

3. The dentist may show the patient the damage to her teeth, and discuss how she feels about herself, while covering the topic of weight loss and the behavior that may be causing the damage.

4. The entire dentition should be examined for decay and sensitivity to hot and cold. The parotid and saliva glands can be examined to evaluate if they are tender and swollen, causing discomfort. The complete oral cavity should be carefully evaluated with special attention to possible sore tissues resulting from poor periodontal health.

TEXTBOOK REVIEW ANSWERS

Multiple Choice

| 1. d | 2. b | 3. d | 4. c | 5. b | 6. a | 7. b | 8.c |

| 9. b | 10. b |

Critical Thinking

1. Knowledge of good nutrition benefits both the dental assistant and patients in providing insight in maintaining overall health.

2. The dental assistant should share the information with the dentist about a patient being bulimic. This information will help the dental team to provide better care for the patient, and the information will be kept confidential. The dentist can discuss the effects of bulimia with the patient and show her or him what happens to the teeth, as well as the effects on the person's overall health.

3. Food labels need to be understood so that individuals can make informed decisions. The labels must cover pertinent information and be understandable. The consumer should be able to determine if the food contains sugar, trans fat, and carbohydrates. The dental assistant can suggest that patients eat foods that will not damage the teeth.

General Anatomy and Physiology

SPECIFIC INSTRUCTIONAL OBJECTIVES

1. List the body systems, body planes and directions, and cavities of the body, and describe the structure and function of the cell.

2. Explain the functions and divisions of the skeletal system, list the composition of the bone, and identify the types of joints.

3. List the functions and parts of the muscular system.

4. List the functions and the structure of the nervous system.

5. List the functions and the parts of the endocrine system.

6. Explain dental concerns related to the reproductive system.

7. Explain the functions of the circulatory system and list and identify the parts.

8. Explain the functions and parts of the digestive system.

9. List the functions and parts of the respiratory system.

10. List the functions and parts of the lymphatic system and the immune system.

11. List the functions and parts of the integumentary system.

PREPARATORY

Personnel

Primary instructor who is knowledgeable about general anatomy, and understands the information that the dental assistant needs to know when caring for dental patients.

Suggested Audiovisual and Resource Materials

Anatomy models

Anatomic charts

DVDs/videos that cover the different body systems

▶ *Workbook:* Chapter 6.

▶ *Image Library:* Provides illustrations from Chapter 6 of the textbook that can be used via computer or as transparencies to provide visual support for classroom instruction.

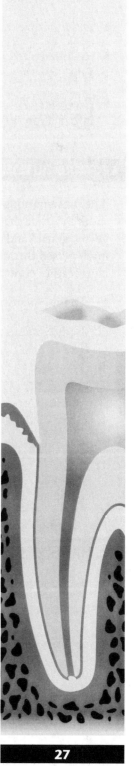

27

▸ *Computerized Test Bank:* Provides additional test questions for Chapter 6.

▸ *CourseMate:* Additional practice exercises that further reinforce Chapter 6 content can be found on the CourseMate Web site.

▸ *Dental Assisting Coloring Book:* Additional practice exercises that further reinforce Chapter 6 content.

▸ *Dental Terminology, Third Edition:* Chapter 2, Anatomy and Oral Structures.

▸ *Delmar's Dental Assisting Exam Review:* Additional review material, test questions, and rationales provide practice for the DANB examination.

▸ *Delmar's Dental Drug Reference:* Provides a detailed review of over 300 drugs and their dental concerns.

▸ *Recommended Reading:* For more detailed information refer to *Body Structures and Functions,* Eleventh Edition.

▸ *Recommended minimum time to complete Chapter 6:* 5 to 10 hours, depending on the depth of information the instructor wishes to cover.

LECTURE OUTLINE CORRELATED TO INSTRUCTOR PRESENTATIONS IN POWERPOINT

The presentations provided contain lecture notes. The notes can be viewed in PowerPoint when viewing the slides in either the normal or outline view. To print the slides with the notes: From your print box look for the "Print What" and change the drop-down to "Notes Pages." A new feature called "Dental Checks" has been interspersed throughout the presentations to keep the student engaged in the materials during the lecture. This feature contains a quick question followed by the answer to stimulate a brief discussion.

1. Define Anatomy and Physiology (Slide 2)

2. Body Systems—list the body systems (Slide 3)

3. Body Planes and Directions (Slides 4 and 5)

   a. Teaching strategy: have the students label the diagrams to review the body planes and directions.

4. Body Cavities (Slide 7)

5. Basic Structure and Functions of the Cell—describe the structure and function of the cell (Slides 8 and 9)

6. Skeletal System—explain the functions and divisions of the skeletal system, list the composition of the bone, and identify the types of joints

   i. Functions of the Skeletal System (Slide 10)

   ii. Divisions of the Skeletal System (Slide 11)

   iii. Composition of the Bones (Slides 12 and 13)

   iv. Types of Joints (Slide 14)

   v. Common Diseases and Conditions of the Skeletal System (Slide 15)

7. Muscular System—list the functions and parts of the muscular system

   i. Functions of the Muscular System (Slide 17)

   ii. Types of Muscles (Slide 18)

      iii. Muscle Characteristics (Slide 19)

      iv. Muscle Attachments (Slide 20)

      v. How Muscles Function (Slide 21)

      vi. Common Conditions and Diseases of the Muscular System (Slides 22 and 23)

8. Nervous System—list the functions and the structure of the nervous system

      i. Functions of the Nervous System (Slide 25)

      ii. Structure of the Nervous System (Slide 26)

      iii. The Spinal Cord and Spinal Nerves (Slide 27)

      iv. The Brain and Cranial Nerves (Slide 28)

      v. Common Diseases of the Nervous System (Slide 29)

9. Endocrine System and Reproductive System—list the functions and the parts of the endocrine system (Slides 31 through 36)

      i. Functions of the Endocrine System

      ii. Parts of the Endocrine System

      iii. Reproductive System—explain the dental concerns related to the reproductive system

      iv. Common Diseases and Conditions of the Endocrine and Reproductive Systems

10. Circulatory System—explain the functions of the circulatory system and list and identify the parts

      i. Functions of the Circulatory System (Slide 37)

      ii. Parts of the Circulatory System (Slides 38 through 45)

      iii. Common Diseases and Conditions of the Circulatory System (Slide 46)

11. Digestive System—explain the functions and parts of the digestive system

      i. Functions of the Digestive System (Slide 48)

      ii. Parts of the Digestive System (Slides 49 and 50)

      iii. Common Diseases and Conditions of the Digestive System (Slide 51)

12. Respiratory System—list the functions and parts of the respiratory system

      i. Functions of the Respiratory System (Slide 52)

      ii. Parts of the Respiratory System (Slide 53)

      iii. Common Diseases of the Respiratory System (Slide 54)

13. Lymphatic System and Immune System—list the functions and parts of the lymphatic system and the immune system

      i. Functions of the Lymphatic System (Slide 56)

      ii. Parts of the Lymphatic System (Slide 57)

iii. Functions of the Immune System (Slide 58)

iv. Common Diseases and Conditions of the Lymphatic and Immune Systems (Slide 59)

14. Integumentary System – list the functions and parts of the integumentary system

i. Functions of the Integumentary System (Slides 60 and 61)

ii. Parts of the Integumentary System (Slide 62)

iii. Abnormal Coloration of the Skin (Slide 63)

iv. Diseases and Conditions of the Integumentary System (Slide 64)

TEACHING STRATEGIES

1. Chapter contents are presented in the PowerPoint slides, which are found in the Instructor Resources to Accompany Delmar's *Dental Assisting*.

2. Much of the content in this chapter is going to have to be remembered by the student and then applied when working on patients in the clinical setting.

3. Have the students research a particular disease, and then arrange group discussions on how the disease/condition affects the patient and what the dental assistant could do to make a dental appointment easier for a patient with this disease.

4. Have the students "build a person." This exercise assists the students with hands-on learning. Each student could build his or her own "person" or the students could be divided into small groups. Each group could be responsible for all the systems or for a single system. This exercise assists in learning the body systems, encourages creativity, and builds teamwork.

CASE STUDY ANSWERS

1. The digestive system (primarily) and muscular system are affected.

2. The alimentary canal: oral cavity, pharynx, esophagus, stomach, and the small and large intestines are the specific structures of the primary system that could be involved.

3. The patient's age and/or medical condition would not specifically impact the situation.

TEXTBOOK REVIEW ANSWERS

Multiple Choice

1. c   2. c   3. a   4. b   5. b   6. c   7. a   8. b

9. d   10. b

Critical Thinking

1. The temporal mandibular joint (TMJ).

2. All arteries of the body carry blood away from the heart; therefore, the vessel going from the heart to the lungs is called an artery. All veins of the body carry blood toward the heart; therefore, the vessel from the lungs to the heart is called a vein. The vessels are named according to their function and not according to whether they carry oxygenated or deoxygenated blood.

3. As a person ages, the yellow bone marrow replaces the red bone marrow. The red bone marrow is where red blood cells are manufactured. Thus, it takes longer to replenish the lost blood.

Head and Neck Anatomy

SPECIFIC INSTRUCTIONAL OBJECTIVES

1. List and identify the landmarks of the face and the oral cavity, including the tongue, floor of the mouth, and salivary glands.

2. Identify the bones of the cranium and the face and identify the landmarks on the maxilla and the mandible.

3. Identify the parts of the temporomandibular joint (TMJ) and describe how the joint works.

4. List and identify the muscles of mastication, facial expression, the floor of the mouth, the tongue, the throat, the neck, and the shoulders. Explain their functions.

5. List and identify the nerves of the maxilla and the mandible.

6. Identify the arteries and veins of the head and the neck.

PREPARATORY

Personnel

Primary instructor who is knowledgeable about head and neck anatomy and understands the information that the dental assistant needs to know and refer to when caring for dental patients.

Suggested Audiovisual and Resource Materials

▶ *Workbook:* Chapter 7.

▶ *Image Library:* Provides illustrations from Chapter 7 of the textbook that can be used via computer to provide visual support for classroom instruction.

▶ *Computerized Test Bank:* Provides additional test questions for Chapter 7 content that can be found on the companion software disk. Refer to models, charts, and DVDs/videos that cover the anatomy of the head and neck areas.

▶ *CourseMate:* Additional practice exercises that further reinforce Chapter 7 content can be found on the CourseMate Web site.

▶ *Dental Assisting Coloring Book:* Additional practice exercises that further reinforce Chapter 7 content.

▶ *Dental Terminology, Third Edition:* Chapter 2, Anatomy and Oral Structures.

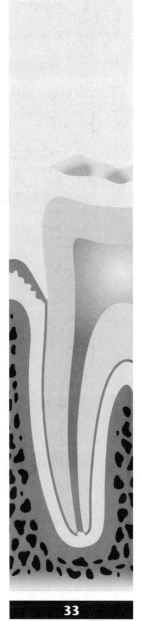

33

▸ *Delmar's Dental Assisting Exam Review:* Additional review material, test questions, and rationale provide practice for the DANB examination.

▸ *Recommended minimum time to complete Chapter* 7: 5 to 6 hours, depending on depth of information the instructor wants to cover.

LECTURE OUTLINE CORRELATED TO INSTRUCTOR PRESENTATIONS IN POWERPOINT

The presentations provided contain lecture notes. The notes can be viewed in PowerPoint when viewing the slides in either the normal or outline view. To print the slides with the notes: From your print box look for the "Print What" and change the drop-down to "Notes Pages." A new feature called "Dental Checks" has been interspersed throughout the presentations to keep the student engaged in the materials during the lecture. This feature contains a quick question followed by the answer to stimulate a brief discussion.

1. Landmarks of the Face and Oral Cavity (Slides 2 through 11)

    i. Landmarks of the Face

    ii. Landmarks of the Oral Cavity

    iii. Palate Area of the Oral Cavity

    iv. Tongue

    v. Floor of the Mouth

    vi. Salivary Glands

    vii. **Teaching Strategy**: Use an intraoral camera to show the various landmarks of the face and oral cavity. Include diagrams for the students to label.

2. Bones of the Head (Slides 13 through 25)

    i. Bones of the Cranium

    ii. Bones of the Face

    iii. **Teaching Strategy**: Use a model of a skull to identify the bones of the cranium and face.

3. Temporomandibular Joint

4. Muscles of the Head and Neck (Slides 26 through 35)

    i. Muscles of Mastication

    ii. Muscles of Facial Expression

    iii. Muscles of the Tongue

    iv. Muscles of the Floor of the Mouth

    v. Muscles of the Soft Palate

    vi. Muscles of the Neck

    vii. **Teaching Strategy**: Have the students locate the muscles on themselves as they are discussed.

5. Nerves of the Head and Neck (Slides 37 through 40)

    i. Maxillary Branch of the Trigeminal Nerve

    ii. Mandibular Branch of the Trigeminal Nerve

6. Circulation of the Head and Neck (Slides 41 through 45)

    i. Arteries of the Face and Oral Cavity

    ii. External Carotid Artery

    iii. Veins of the Face and Oral Cavity

TEACHING STRATEGIES

1. Chapter contents are presented in the PowerPoint slides in the Electronic Classroom Manager to Accompany Delmar's *Dental Assisting*.

2. Much of the content in this chapter is going to have to be remembered by the student and then applied in the clinical setting.

3. Have the students research a disease that affects each area of the head and neck that is discussed, and then arrange group discussions on how the disease/condition affects the patient and what the dental assistant could do to make a dental appointment easier for this patient.

4. Have the students continue to "build a person." Each student could add on to his or her own person or to the person built in a small group. The students could be responsible for all areas or for just one to complete this project. This exercise helps students learn head and neck anatomy, encourages creativity, and builds teamwork.

CASE STUDY ANSWERS

1. Primarily the temporomandibular joint (TMJ) area, including the glenoid fossa of the temporal bone, the articular eminence of the temporal bone, the condyloid process of the mandible, the articular disc, and a dense fibrous capsule containing the synovial fluid are the components of the head and neck affected.

2. The disc in the TMJ can become displaced or stuck, causing more severe problems as time passes.

3. The dental assistant can review the health history, notify the dentist, and note the symptoms on the patient's chart.

TEXTBOOK REVIEW ANSWERS

Multiple Choice

1. c	2. d	3. b	4. b	5. b	6. b	7. a
8. c	9. a	10. d				

Critical Thinking

1. Right middle superior alveolar nerve.

2. This facial landmark is called the philtrum. The developmental disturbance that can occur is a cleft lip (unilateral or bilateral).

3. Torso palatinus, found on the center of the palate. Torus mandibularis, found on the lingual side of the mandible, near the canines and premolars.

Embryology and Histology

SPECIFIC INSTRUCTIONAL OBJECTIVES

1. Identify the terms and times of the three phases of pregnancy.

2. Describe how the human face develops and changes during the zygote and embryo phases.

3. Describe the life cycle of a tooth and identify the stages.

4. Identify the four primary structures of the tooth and the location and function of each.

5. Identify the substances of enamel, dentin, cementum, and pulp and their identifying marks.

6. Identify the components of the periodontium and the considerations of the alveolar bone.

7. Describe the structures of the gingiva and the mucosa.

PREPARATORY

Personnel

Primary instructor who is knowledgeable about embryology and histology. It is recommended that the same instructor teach tooth anatomy and morphology, as these topics build on current chapter content.

Suggested Audiovisual and Resource Materials

A number of videos are available on embryology. Many video stores stock *The Miracle of Life* (Nova), which shows the development of life and how the face develops and changes during the zygote and embryo phases.

▶ *Workbook:* Chapter 8.

▶ *Image Library:* Provides illustrations from Chapter 8 of the textbook that can be used via computer or as transparencies to provide visual support for classroom instruction.

▶ *Computerized Test Bank:* Provides additional test questions for Chapter 8 and related material on the DANB examination.

▶ *Practice Software:* Additional practice exercises that further reinforce Chapter 8 content can be found on the companion software disk.

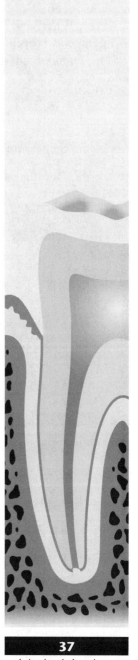

▶ *CourseMate:* Additional practice exercises that further reinforce Chapter 8 content can be found on the CourseMate Web site.

▶ *Dental Assisting Coloring Book:* Additional practice exercises that further reinforce Chapter 8 content.

▶ *Dental Terminology, Third Edition:* Chapter 3, Tooth Origin and Formation.

▶ *Delmar's Dental Assisting Exam Review:* Additional review material, test questions, and rationale provide practice for the DANB examination.

▶ *Recommended minimum time to complete Chapter 8:* 4 hours, depending on depth of information the instructor wishes to cover.

LECTURE OUTLINE CORRELATED TO INSTRUCTOR PRESENTATIONS IN POWERPOINT

The presentations provided contain lecture notes. The notes can be viewed in PowerPoint when viewing the slides in either the normal or outline view. To print the slides with the notes: From your print box look for the "Print What" and change the drop-down to "Notes Pages." A new feature called "Dental Checks" has been interspersed throughout the presentations to keep the student engaged in the materials during the lecture. This feature contains a quick question followed by the answer to stimulate a brief discussion.

1. Embryology (Slides 2 through 4)

   i. Primitive Facial Development (Slide 5)

   ii. Stages and Features of Pregnancy (Slide 6)

   iii. Developmental Disturbances (Slides 7 through 11)

2. Histology and the Life Cycle of the Tooth (Slides 13 through 16)

   i. Bud Stage

   ii. Cap Stage

   iii. Bell Stage

   iv. Maturation Stage

3. Tooth Structure (Slides 17 through 25)

   i. Enamel

   ii. Dentin

   iii. Pulp

4. Components of the Periodontium (Slides 27 through 34)

   i. Cementum

   ii. Alveolar Bone

   iii. Periodontal Ligament

   iv. Gingiva

TEACHING STRATEGIES

1. Chapter contents are presented in the PowerPoint slides, which are found in the Instructor Resources that accompany *Dental Assisting: A Comprehensive Approach*, *4th edition*.

2. Videos on embryology can be shown to break up the lecture. Videos (e.g., *The Miracle of Life*) can be obtained from the school library or elsewhere.

3. A quiz or a Web assignment can be required of the students to again review the material and broaden their knowledge base.

CASE STUDY ANSWERS

1. The permanent teeth erupt and apply pressure to the apex of the roots of the primary teeth. During this force, osteoclasts, or bone resorption cells, will evanesce, or dissolve, the root of the primary tooth. This resorption will first take place at the apex, and then continue up toward the crown of the tooth.

2. The periodontal fibers that may remain attached at this stage, assuming that the primary tooth root has been resorbed, are the alveolar crest fibers, the horizontal fiber group, and the oblique fiber.

3. The primary teeth occupy and maintain space in the dental arches for the permanent teeth and act as a guide during the eruption process. If the tooth is early, the space may be diminished, causing crowding when the permanent teeth erupt.

TEXTBOOK REVIEW ANSWERS

Multiple Choice

1. a   2. a   3. a   4. d   5. b   6. b   7. d

8. a   9. d   10. b

Critical Thinking

1. Based on statistics only, the child would most probably be male. The child's parents should be given information related to cleft palate. This information should include names and contact information of medical and dental professionals who handle this type of case, names of Web sites the parents may be able to go to find additional information on the condition, as well as the names of any support groups in the area. The baby's nursing and feeding needs will need to be addressed.

2. Cycle, apposition; stage, maturation.

3. They would present a problem for endodontic treatment. The calcified masses of dentin material are called pulp stones.

CHAPTER 9

Tooth Morphology

SPECIFIC INSTRUCTIONAL OBJECTIVES

1. Identify the dental arches and quadrants using the correct terminology.

2. List the primary and permanent teeth by name and location.

3. Explain the eruption schedule for the primary and permanent teeth.

4. Identify the different divisions of the tooth, including clinical and anatomical divisions.

5. Identify the surfaces of each tooth and their locations.

6. List the anatomical structures and their definitions.

7. Describe each permanent tooth according to location, anatomical features, morphology, function, position, and other identifying factors.

8. Describe each deciduous (primary) tooth according to its location, anatomical features, morphology, function, position, and other identifying factors.

PREPARATORY

Personnel

Primary instructor who is knowledgeable about tooth development and morphology. It is advisable that the instructor who teaches histology also teaches tooth morphology.

Suggested Audiovisual and Resource Materials

Several videos are available on tooth morphology.

▶ *Workbook:* Chapter 9.

▶ *Image Library:* Provides illustrations from Chapter 9 of the textbook that can be used via computer or as transparencies to provide visual support for classroom instruction.

▶ *Computerized Test Bank:* Provides additional test questions for Chapter 9 and related material on the DANB examination.

▶ *Practice Software:* Additional practice exercises that further reinforce Chapter 9 content can be found on the companion software disk.

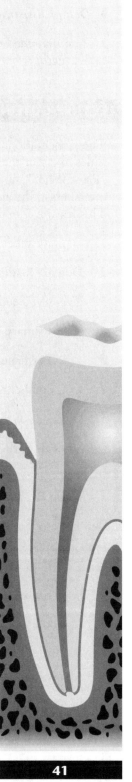

▶ *Dental Terminology, Third Edition:* Chapter 3, Tooth Origin and Formation.

▶ *Delmar's Dental Assisting Exam Review:* Additional review material, test questions, and rationale provide practice for the DANB examination.

▶ *Delmar's Dental Drug Reference:* Provides a detailed review of over 300 drugs and their dental concerns.

▶ *CourseMate:* Additional practice exercises that further reinforce Chapter 9 content can be found on the CourseMate Web site.

▶ *Dental Assisting Coloring Book:* Additional practice exercises that further reinforce Chapter 9 content.

▶ *Recommended minimum time to complete Chapter 9:* 6 hours, depending on depth of information the instructor wishes to cover.

LECTURE OUTLINE CORRELATED TO INSTRUCTOR PRESENTATIONS IN POWERPOINT

The presentations provided contain lecture notes. The notes can be viewed in PowerPoint when viewing the slides in either the normal or outline view. To print the slides with the notes: From your print box look for the "Print What" and change the drop-down to "Notes Pages." A new feature called "Dental Checks" has been interspersed throughout the presentations to keep the student engaged in the materials during the lecture. This feature contains a quick question followed by the answer to stimulate a brief discussion.

1. Dental Arches (Slide 2)

2. Dental Quadrants (Slides 3 and 4)

3. Types of Teeth and Their Functions (Slides 5 through 8)

    i. Primary Teeth

    ii. Permanent Teeth

4. Eruption Schedule (Slide 9)

5. Divisions of the Tooth (Slide 10)

6. Surfaces of the Teeth (Slides 11 through 17)

    i. Anterior Teeth

    ii. Posterior Teeth

    iii. Contact

    iv. Diastema

    v. Embrasure

7. Anatomical Structures (Slides 18 through 28)

8. Permanent Teeth (Slides 29 through 50)

    i. Maxillary Central Incisor

    ii. Maxillary Lateral Incisor

    iii. Maxillary Canine (Cuspid)

      iv. Maxillary First Premolar (Bicuspid)

      v. Maxillary Second Premolar (Bicuspid)

      vi. Maxillary First Molar

      vii. Maxillary Second Molar

      viii. Maxillary Third Molar

      ix. Mandibular Central Incisor

      x. Mandibular Lateral Incisor

      xi. Mandibular Canine (Cuspid)

      xii. Mandibular First Premolar (Bicuspid)

      xiii. Mandibular Second Premolar (Bicuspid)

      xiv. Mandibular Molars

      xv. Mandibular First Molar

      xvi. Mandibular Second Molar

      xvii. Mandibular Third Molar

9. Deciduous (Primary) Teeth Descriptions (Slides 51 through 71)

      i. Maxillary Deciduous Central Incisor

      ii. Maxillary Deciduous Lateral Incisor

      iii. Maxillary Deciduous Canine (Cuspid)

      iv. Maxillary Deciduous First Molar

      v. Maxillary Deciduous Second Molar

      vi. Mandibular Deciduous Central Incisor

      vii. Mandibular Deciduous Lateral Incisor

      viii. Mandibular Deciduous Canine (Cuspid)

      ix. Mandibular Deciduous First Molar

      x. Mandibular Deciduous Second Molar

TEACHING STRATEGIES

1. Chapter contents are presented in the PowerPoint slides, which are found in the Instructor Resources to Accompany Delmar's *Dental Assisting*.

2. Videos on tooth morphology can be shown to break up the lecture. Although videos are useful, most of this content can be visualized well by studying models of the oral cavity.

3. A quiz or a Web assignment can be required of students to again review the material and broaden their knowledge base.

4. One of the best ways for students to study tooth morphology is to have models of the teeth to handle and examine. Models can be purchased, or made in the laboratory (but not by the students currently being introduced to morphology). Many schools include pouring of plaster models from rubber molds in the laboratory portion of the program.

5. When discussing the names and numbers of the teeth, consider having master sheets available that show all of the teeth (such as Figure 9-4) but do not include names. Have each student label each tooth and number it according to the universal numbering system.

CASE STUDY ANSWERS

1. It is probable that the second permanent molars are beginning to erupt through the tissue.

2. The dental assistant should ask about the level and frequency of the patient's discomfort. Travis should not be concerned, because the discomfort is a normal part of the eruption process.

3. The dental assistant should ask what brings on the discomfort. Travis would not expect primary tooth loss in these areas, because a second permanent molar would come in behind the primary dentition.

TEXTBOOK REVIEW ANSWERS

Multiple Choice

1. c   2. b   3. c   4. b   5. d   6. b   7. c

8. a   9. d   10. a

Critical Thinking

1. The mandibular deciduous first molar would be retained in the place of the mandibular first bicuspid (premolar).

2. The maxillary first bicuspids are the bifurcated teeth in the maxillary arch.

3. The facial, or labial, surface is convex on the anterior teeth.

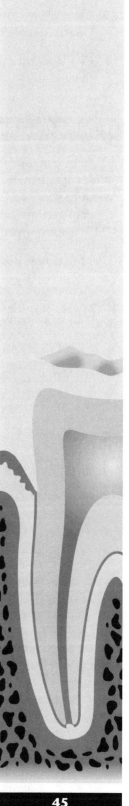

CHAPTER 10

Microbiology

SPECIFIC INSTRUCTIONAL OBJECTIVES

1. Identify Anton Van Leeuwenhoek, Ferdinand Cohn, Louis Pasteur, Robert Koch, and Richard Petri according to their contributions to microbiology.

2. Explain the groups of microorganisms and staining procedures used to identify them.

3. Identify the characteristics pertaining to bacteria.

4. List the characteristics of protozoa.

5. Identify the characteristics of *Rickettsia*.

6. Explain the characteristics of yeasts and molds.

7. List the characteristics of viruses.

8. Describe the diseases of major concern to the dental assistant and explain why they cause concern.

9. Identify how the body fights disease. Explain types of immunities and routes of microorganism infection.

PREPARATORY

Personnel

Primary instructor who is knowledgeable about microbiology. It is advisable that the instructor has background knowledge in dental infection control.

Suggested Audiovisual and Resource Materials

Several videos on microbiology fundamentals are available. Many supplemental videos on disease-producing microorganisms are available in school and public libraries.

▶ *Workbook:* Chapter 10.

▶ *Image Library:* Provides illustrations from Chapter 10 of the textbook that can be used via computer or as transparencies to provide visual support for classroom instruction.

▶ *Computerized Test Bank:* Provides additional test questions for Chapter 10 and related material on the DANB examination.

▶ *Practice Software:* Additional practice exercises that further reinforce Chapter 10 content can be found on the companion software disk.

▶ *Dental Terminology, Third Edition:* Chapter 5, Infection Control.

▶ *Delmar's Dental Assisting Exam Review:* Additional review material, test questions, and rationales provide practice for the DANB examination.

▶ *CourseMate:* Additional practice exercises that further reinforce Chapter 10 content can be found on the CourseMate Web site.

▶ *Recommended minimum time to complete Chapter 10:* 5 to 7 hours, depending on depth of information the instructor wishes to cover.

LECTURE OUTLINE CORRELATED TO INSTRUCTOR PRESENTATIONS IN POWERPOINT

The presentations provided contain lecture notes. The notes can be viewed in PowerPoint when viewing the slides in either the normal or outline view. To print the slides with the notes: From your print box look for the "Print What" and change the drop-down to "Notes Pages." A new feature called "Dental Checks" has been interspersed throughout the presentations to keep the student engaged in the materials during the lecture. This feature contains a quick question followed by the answer to stimulate a brief discussion.

1. Important People in Microbiology (Slides 2 through 5)

    i. Anton Van Leeuwenhoek

    ii. Ferdinand Julius Cohn

    iii. Louis Pasteur

    iv. Robert Koch

    v. Richard Julius Petri

2. Groups of Microorganisms (Slide 6)

3. Bacteria (Slides 7 through 14)

    i. Bacteria's Need for Oxygen

    ii. The Morphology of Bacteria

    iii. Examples of Diseases Caused by Bacteria

        a. Tuberculosis

        b. Legionellosis

        c. Diphtheria, pertussis, and tetanus

        d. Strep throat

        e. Staphylococcal infections

        f. Anthrax

        g. Chlamydiae

4. Protozoa (Slides 16 through 19)

   i. Examples of Diseases Caused by Protozoa

      a. Amebic dysentery

      b. Periodontal disease

      c. Malaria

5. Rickettsiae (Slides 20 through 22)

   i. Examples of Diseases Caused by Rickettsiae

      a. Rocky Mountain Spotted Fever

      b. Typhus

      c. Head Lice

6. Yeasts and Molds (Slides 23 through 25)

   i. Examples of Diseases Caused by Yeasts and Molds

      a. Candidiasis

      b. Tinea

7. Prions (Slide 26)

   i. Mad Cow Disease

   ii. Creutzfeldt-Jakob Disease

8. Viruses (Slides 27 through 34)

   i. Examples of Diseases Caused by Viruses

      a. Measles, mumps, and rubella

      b. Epstein-Barr

      c. Mononucleosis

      d. West Nile Virus

      e. Poliomyelitis

      f. Chickenpox

      g. Common cold and influenza

9. Diseases of Major Concern to the Dental Assistant (Slides 36 through 41)

   i. Herpes Simplex

   ii. Viral Hepatitis

   iii. Human Immunodeficiency Virus

   iv. Acquired Immunodeficiency Syndrome

10. How the Body Resists Diseases (Slides 43 through 47)

     i. Infection

    ii. Immunity

TEACHING STRATEGIES

1. Chapter contents are presented in the PowerPoint slides, which are found in the Electronic Classroom Manager to Accompany Delmar's *Dental Assisting*.

2. Videos on microbiology can be shown to break up the lecture.

3. A quiz or a Web assignment can be required of the students to again review the material and broaden their knowledge base.

4. If the instructor works with the biology lab at the school, each student can take a sample in an area of the lab where bacteria is suspected and place it in a Petri dish to watch for growth of microorganisms.

5. Have the students research microorganisms in the news, and have them complete a one-page paper.

CASE STUDY ANSWERS

1. You would consider Rocky Mountain spotted fever.

2. Rocky Mountain spotted fever is an uncommon disease.

3. Treatment with antibiotic drugs normally cures the disease.

4. Rickettsiae caused the disease.

TEXTBOOK REVIEW ANSWERS

Multiple Choice

1. c   2. a   3. d   4. b   5. a   6. b   7. b

8. c   9. b   10. c

Critical Thinking

1. No, the probability is not high for the other individual to acquire AIDS or HIV.

2. Bacteria and protozoa can be associated with periodontal disease.

3. Hepatitis B, because it is primarily transmitted through contaminated needles and syringes.

CHAPTER 11

Infection Control

SPECIFIC INSTRUCTIONAL OBJECTIVES

1. Identify the rationale, regulations, recommendations, and training that govern infection control in the dental office.

2. Describe how pathogens travel from person to person in the dental office.

3. List the three primary routes of microbial transmission and the associated dental procedures that affect the dental assistant.

4. Demonstrate the principles of infection control, including medical history, handwashing, personal protective equipment, barriers, chemical disinfectants, ultrasonic cleaners, sterilizers, and instrument storage.

5. List various disinfectants and their applications as used in dentistry.

6. Identify and demonstrate the usage of different types of sterilizers.

7. Demonstrate the usage of several types of sterilization monitors, such as biological and process indicators.

8. Identify and show the proper usage of preprocedure mouth rinses, high-volume evacuation, dental dams, and disposable items.

9. Identify and demonstrate the correct protocol for disinfecting, cleaning, and sterilizing prior to seating the patient, as well as at the end of the dental treatment, in the dental radiography area, and in the dental laboratory.

PREPARATORY

Personnel

Primary instructor who is knowledgeable about infection control in the dental office. It is advisable that the instructor has background knowledge in microbiology as well.

Suggested Audiovisual and Resource Materials

Several videos are available on dental office infection control.

▶ *Workbook:* Chapter 11.

▶ *Delmar's Dental Assisting Video Series:* Appropriate content is available on Tape 3, *Infection Control Techniques.* This includes the donning of PPE, handwashing, preparation of the dental treatment room, completion of treatment, disinfection of the treatment room following treatment, and treatment of contaminated tray and equipment in the sterilization area.

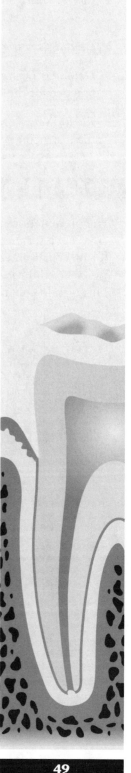

▶ *Image Library:* Provides illustrations from Chapter 11 of the textbook that can be used via computer or as transparencies to provide visual support for classroom instruction.

▶ *Computerized Test Bank:* Provides additional test questions for Chapter 11 and related material on the DANB examination.

▶ *Practice Software:* Additional practice exercises that further reinforce Chapter 11 content can be found on the companion software disk.

▶ *CourseMate:* Additional practice exercises that further reinforce Chapter 11 content can be found on the CourseMate Web site.

▶ *Dental Terminology, Third Edition:* Chapter 5, Infection Control.

▶ *Delmar's Dental Assisting Exam Review:* Additional review material, test questions, and rationales provide practice for the DANB examination.

▶ *Recommended minimum time to complete Chapter 11:* 8 to 10 hours, depending on depth of information the instructor wishes to cover and the time allotted in the laboratory.

LECTURE OUTLINE CORRELATED TO INSTRUCTOR PRESENTATIONS IN POWERPOINT

The presentations provided contain lecture notes. The notes can be viewed in PowerPoint when viewing the slides in either the normal or outline view. To print the slides with the notes: From your print box look for the "Print What" and change the drop-down to "Notes Pages." A new feature called "Dental Checks" has been interspersed throughout the presentations to keep the student engaged in the materials during the lecture. This feature contains a quick question followed by the answer to stimulate a brief discussion.

1. Rationales and Regulations of Infection Control (Slides 2 through 4)

    i. Regulations and Recommendations for Infection Control in the Dental Office

    ii. OSHA-Mandated Training for Dental Office Employees (Slides 5 through 7)

2. Cross-Contamination Pathways (Slide 9)

3. Chain of Infection (Slides 10 through 14)

    i. Agent

    ii. Reservoir

    iii. Portal of Exit

    iv. Mode of Transmission

    v. Portal of Entry

    vi. Host

4. Breaking the Chain of Infection (Slides 15 through 20)

    i. Between Agent and Reservoir

    ii. Between Reservoir and Portal of Exit

    iii. Between Portal of Exit and Mode of Transmission

      iv. Between Mode of Transmission and Portal of Entry

      v. Between Portal of Entry and Host

      vi. Between Host and Agent

5. Routes of Microbial Transmission in the Dental Office (Slide 22)

6. Infection Control in the Dental Office (Slides 23 and 24)

      i. Immunizations

      ii. Medical History

      iii. Handwashing

      iv. Alcohol-Based Hand Rubs

      v. Lotions

      vi. Personal Protective Equipment

      vii. Barriers

7. Disinfection (Slides 25 through 29)

      i. Cleaning the Area

      ii. Environmental Protection Agency Approval

      iii. Chemical Disinfectants

      iv. Disinfection Technique

      v. Ultrasonic Cleaning

      vi. Washer-Disinfector Devices

8. Sterilization (Slides 30 and 31)

      i. Liquid Chemical Disinfectant/Sterilization

      ii. Ethylene Oxide Sterilization

      iii. Dry Heat Sterilization

      iv. Chemical Vapor Sterilization

      v. Steam Under Pressure Sterilization

      vi. Steam Autoclave (Flash) Sterilization

      vii. Equipment Maintenance

      viii. Handpiece Sterilization

      ix. Packaging and Loading Sterilizers

      x. Instrument Storage

9. Sterilization Monitoring (Slide 32)

   i. Biological Monitors

   ii. Process Indicators

   iii. Dosage Indicators

10. Techniques and Aids for Infection Control (Slide 33)

   i. Preprocedure Antiseptic Mouth Rinses

   ii. High-Volume Evacuation

   iii. Dental Dam Usage

   iv. Disposable Items

11. Clinical Asepsis Protocol (Slide 35)

   i. Treatment Area Protocol for Disinfecting and Cleaning (Slides 36 through 38)

12. Dental Unit Waterlines (Slide 39)

13. Dental Radiography Room and Equipment (Slide 40)

14. Dental Laboratory (Slide 41)

TEACHING STRATEGIES

1. Chapter contents are presented in the PowerPoint slides, which are found in the Instructor Resources to Accompany Delmar's *Dental Assisting*.

2. Videos on microbiology can be shown to break up the lecture along with PowerPoint information.

3. A quiz or a Web assignment can be required of the students to again review the material and broaden their knowledge base.

4. Have students wash hands with a handwashing powder, and then use an ultraviolet light to view the residue. This demonstrates for the students missed areas during handwashing. Another activity involves having students with contaminated hands (after washing) shake hands with others, and then view cross-contamination under the light.

CASE STUDY ANSWERS

1. No areas were contaminated if nothing was touched with the contaminated gloves. If Lisa had not removed her gloves, the telephone, telephone book, and sterilization area would have been contaminated.

2. Lisa should have washed her hands after removing her gloves as a further precaution.

3. Lisa used latex or vinyl treatment gloves, and could have used overgloves to cover the latex or vinyl while taking the telephone message. Lisa should have used utility gloves in the sterilization area, and, when returning to the treatment room, she should have donned treatment gloves.

TEXTBOOK REVIEW ANSWERS

Multiple Choice

1. b   2. d   3. a   4. c   5. a   6. d   7. b

8. d   9. b   10. d

Critical Thinking

1. Probably not, because random inspections by OSHA occur in offices with 11 or more employees.

2. Due to the misuse, the liability lies with the user. If the solution had not been misused, the manufacturer would be responsible for problems.

3. Inhalation/aerosol.

Management of Hazardous Materials

SPECIFIC INSTRUCTIONAL OBJECTIVES

1. Identify the scope of the OSHA Bloodborne/Hazardous Materials Standard.

2. Identify physical equipment and mechanical devices provided to safeguard employees.

3. Demonstrate safe disposal of sharps.

4. Describe MSDS manuals.

5. Demonstrate the use of the colors and numbers in hazardous chemical identifcation.

6. Describe employee training required to meet the OSHA standard for hazardous chemicals.

PREPARATORY

Personnel

Primary instructor who is knowledgeable about infection control and the OSHA standard. It is advisable that the instructor has background knowledge in microbiology as well. This instructor must keep updated information on the OSHA standard and what is being done in the workplace to comply with changes.

Suggested Audiovisual and Resource Materials

Several videos are available on hazardous materials and the OSHA standard, including from professional organizations, especially the American Dental Association. Seminars are ongoing on this topic and often have videos and other supplements that can be purchased to enhance classroom teaching of this topic.

▶ *Workbook:* Chapter 12.

▶ *Image Library:* Provides illustrations from Chapter 12 of the textbook that can be used via computer or as transparencies to provide visual support for classroom instruction.

▶ *Computerized Test Bank:* Provides additional test questions for Chapter 12 and related material on the DANB examination.

▶ *Practice Software:* Additional practice exercises that further reinforce Chapter 12 content can be found on the companion software disk.

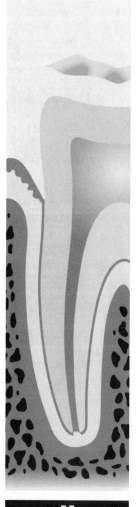

▶ *Dental Terminology, Third Edition:* Chapter 5, Infection Control.

▶ *Delmar's Dental Assisting Exam Review:* Additional review material, test questions, and rationales provide practice for the DANB examination.

▶ *CourseMate:* Additional practice exercises that further reinforce Chapter 12 content can be found on the CourseMate Web site.

▶ *Recommended minimum time to complete Chapter 12:* 3 to 4 hours, depending on depth of information the instructor wishes to cover.

LECTURE OUTLINE CORRELATED TO INSTRUCTOR PRESENTATIONS IN POWERPOINT

The presentations provided contain lecture notes. The notes can be viewed in PowerPoint when viewing the slides in either the normal or outline view. To print the slides with the notes: From your print box look for the "Print What" and change the drop-down to "Notes Pages." A new feature called "Dental Checks" has been interspersed throughout the presentations to keep the student engaged in the materials during the lecture. This feature contains a quick question followed by the answer to stimulate a brief discussion.

1. OSHA's Bloodborne Pathogen Standard (Slides 2 through 29)

    a. Scope and application

    b. Methods of compliance

    c. Standard precautions

    d. Engineering controls

    e. Sharps containers

    f. Workplace controls and rules

    g. Personal protective equipment

    h. Eye protection

    i. Gloves

    j. Protective clothing

    k. Housekeeping

    l. Regulated waste containers

    m. Laundry

    n. Hepatitis B vaccination

    o. Post-exposure follow-up

    p. Labels

    q. Information and training

    r. Training components

    s. Medical records

    t. Training records

    u. Exposure control plan

    v. Employee responsibilities

2. Revision (Slides 31 and 32)

    a. Exposure Control Plan Additions

    b. OSHA Compliance Directive

3. Engineering/Work Practice Controls (Slide 33)

4. Sharps (Slides 34 and 35)

    a. Occupational Exposure to Bloodborne Pathogens (Slide 36)

    b. Employee Work Site

5. Hazardous Chemicals (Slides 37 and 38)

    a. Material Safety Data Sheets (Slide 39)

    b. Chemical warning labels (Slide 40)

TEACHING STRATEGIES

1. Chapter contents are presented in the PowerPoint slides, which are found in the Instructor Resources to Accompany Delmar's *Dental Assisting*.

2. Videos on the management of hazardous materials can be shown to break up the lecture along with PowerPoint slides.

3. A quiz or a Web assignment can be required of the students to again review the material and broaden their knowledge base.

CASE STUDY ANSWERS

1. Rebecca must have had the training on the OSHA Bloodborne/Hazardous Materials Standard within 30 days of employment.

2. Training records must be kept for 3 years from date of training and must include the following:

Date of training

Summary of contents of training program

Name and qualifcations of trainer

Name and job title of all persons attending

Medical records must be kept for each employee with occupational exposure and include (if Rebecca was cut during the removal of this glass, it would be noted in this log): copy of employee's vaccination status and date, copy of postexposure follow-up evaluation procedures, and health care professional's written opinions.

Confidentiality must be maintained.

Records must be maintained for 30 years plus the duration of employment.

3. Rebecca would use a broom and dustpan to pick up the glass. She should not touch it with bare hands. If the glass container held a contaminated substance, Rebecca would use appropriate personal protective equipment (PPE) and follow established protocols to remove the broken glass and decontaminate the exposed surfaces.

4. The glass is placed in a closable, leakproof, puncture-resistant, labeled or color-coded, regulated waste container (sharps container).

TEXTBOOK REVIEW ANSWERS

Multiple Choice

1. c	2. b	3. c	4. d	5. a	6. b	7. d	8. a

9. c   10. c

Critical Thinking

1. No, the employee would be covered under the standard only while at the workplace.

2. Under the OSHA standard, the employer is ultimately responsible.

3. Standard precautions are issued by the Centers for Disease Control and Prevention. They are used to protect the patients and health care workers.

CHAPTER 13

Preparation for Patient Care

SPECIFIC INSTRUCTIONAL OBJECTIVES

1. Explain how the patient record is developed and the importance of the personal registration form, medical and dental information, clinical evaluation, and the extraoral and intraoral examinations.

2. Describe how the patient record may be called into litigation or used in a forensic case.

3. Perform or assist the dentist in an extraoral and an intraoral evaluation including lips, tongue, glands, and oral cavity.

4. Explain how a diagnosis and treatment plan is developed.

5. Perform vital signs on the patient, including both oral and tympanic temperature, pulse, respiration, and blood pressure.

6. Document the vital signs and be alert to any signs that are abnormal.

7. Identify the five Korotkoff sounds, the two that are used in recording blood pressure, and the man who described them in 1905.

PREPARATORY

Personnel

Primary instructor who is knowledgeable about how to prepare the patient for care in the dental office. The instructor should be proficient in performing vital sign readings and in assisting the dentist in an oral evaluation.

Suggested Audiovisual and Resource Materials

Videos on vital sign readings are available. The most difficult part for students is the auditory part. Videos that feature sounds during the taking of blood pressure are helpful. If not, the instructor should obtain a stethoscope with two earpieces, one for the instructor and one for the student to aid the latter in identifying the correct sounds.

▶ *Workbook:* Chapter 13.

▶ *Image Library:* Provides illustrations from Chapter 13 of the textbook that can be used via computer or as transparencies to provide visual support for classroom instruction.

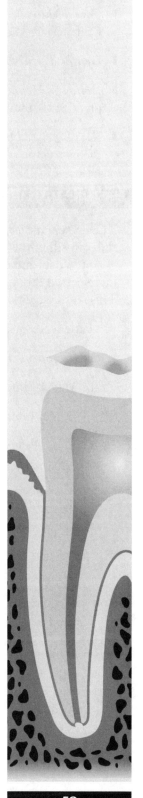

▶ *Computerized Test Bank:* Provides additional test questions for Chapter 13 and related material on the DANB examination.

▶ *Practice Software:* Additional practice exercises that further reinforce Chapter 13 content can be found on the companion software disk.

▶ *Interactive Skills CD:* Taking and Recording Vital Signs.

▶ *CourseMate:* Additional practice exercises that further reinforce Chapter 13 content can be found on the CourseMate Web site.

▶ *Dental Terminology, Third Edition:* Chapter 7, Examination and Prevention.

▶ *Delmar's Dental Assisting Exam Review:* Additional review material, test questions, and rationales provide practice for the DANB examination.

▶ *Recommended minimum time to complete Chapter 13:* 3 to 4 hours, depending on depth of information the instructor wishes to cover.

LECTURE OUTLINE CORRELATED TO INSTRUCTOR PRESENTATIONS IN POWERPOINT

The presentations provided contain lecture notes. The notes can be viewed in PowerPoint when viewing the slides in either the normal or outline view. To print the slides with the notes: From your print box look for the "Print What" and change the drop-down to "Notes Pages." A new feature called "Dental Checks" has been interspersed throughout the presentations to keep the student engaged in the materials during the lecture. This feature contains a quick question followed by the answer to stimulate a brief discussion.

1. Patient Record (Slide 2)

    a. Personal Information (Slide 3)

    b. Medical Information (Slide 4)

    c. Dental Information (Slide 5)

2. Clinical Observation and Physical Assessment (Slide 6)

    a. Gait

    b. Behavior

    c. Speech

    d. Facial symmetry

    e. Eyes and skin

3. Clinical Setting (Slide 7)

    a. Signing of consent forms

    b. Referral information

    c. Taking of radiographs if necessary

4. Clinical Evaluation (Slides 8 through 17)

    a. Mouth and lips

    b. Mandible and floor of mouth

      c. Cervical lymph nodes

      d. Temporomandibular joint

      e. Floor of mouth

      f. Mucosa and frenum

      g. Tongue and palate

5. Diagnosis and Treatment Plan (Slide 19)

6. Vital Signs (Slide 20)

      a. Body Temperature (Slide 21)

         i. Oral or tympanic

         ii. Antipyretic

         iii. Hypothermic

      b. Pulse (Slides 22 through 24)

         i. Pulse sites

         ii. Characteristics

         iii. Tachycardia vs bradycardia

      c. Respiration (Slides 25 and 26)

         i. Inhalation and exhalation

         ii. Rate and depth

         iii. Tachypnea vs bradypnea

      d. Blood Pressure (Slides 27 through 32)

         i. Systolic and diastolic

         ii. Korotkoff sounds

         iii. Hypertension vs hypotension

         iv. Palpation vs auscultation

TEACHING STRATEGIES

1. Chapter contents are presented in the PowerPoint slides, which are found in the Instructor Resources to Accompany Delmar's *Dental Assisting*.

2. Videos on the skills of performing vital signs on patients can be shown to break up the lecture with Power-Point slides.

3. A quiz or a Web assignment can be required of the students to again review the material and broaden their knowledge base.

CASE STUDY ANSWERS

1. Dwayne's blood pressure does not fall within the normal range because the systolic pressure is above 140.

2. The blood pressure should be retaken to ensure that it was accurate.

3. This reading should be brought to the attention of the dentist.

TEXTBOOK REVIEW ANSWERS

Multiple Choice

1. c   2. a   3. d   4. b   5. d   6. d   7. b   8. b

9. a   10. c

Critical Thinking

1. Any temperature over 99.5° F is a fever. Discuss with the dentist that the patient has a high temperature. Decisions can be made to reschedule the patient or to complete the scheduled treatment, depending on the situation.

2. The patient may be nervous and unsettled before and during dental treatment. The dental assistant can listen to the patient's concerns, explain the procedure, and give reassurances.

3. Discuss this with the patient. It may have been as simple as a leg falling asleep while the patient waited to be seated in the treatment room, or it may be something he or she did not put down on the medical history, believing that it has no relevance to the dental treatment. Remember that the more thorough the information, the better the dental team is able to provide services.

Dental Charting

SPECIFIC INSTRUCTIONAL OBJECTIVES

1. Explain why charting is used in dental practices.

2. Identify charts that use symbols to represent conditions in the oral cavity.

3. List and explain the systems used for charting the permanent and deciduous dentitions.

4. Define G.V. Black's six classifications of cavity preparations.

5. List common abbreviations used to identify simple, compound, and complex cavities.

6. Describe basic dental charting terminology.

7. Explain color indicators and identify charting symbols.

PREPARATORY

Personnel

Primary instructor who is knowledgeable about dental assisting, especially chairside assisting and dental charting. The instructor should also have a background in tooth morphology and head and neck anatomy.

Suggested Audiovisual and Resource Materials

▶ *Workbook:* Chapter 14.

▶ *Transparencies:*

Transparency Master 34—(A) Universal/National numbering and lettering system.

(B) Computer charting done with the Universal numbering and lettering system.

Transparency Master 35—International Standards Organization (ISO) TC 10; Designation System/Fédération Dentaire International System.

Transparency Master 36—Palmer numbering and lettering system.

▶ *Image Library:* Provides illustrations from Chapter 14 of the textbook that can be used via computer or as transparencies to provide visual support for classroom instruction.

▶ *Computerized Test Bank:* Provides additional test questions for Chapter 14 and related material on the DANB examination.

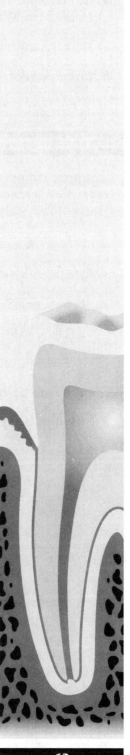

▶ *Practice Software:* Additional practice exercises that further reinforce Chapter 14 content can be found on the companion software disk.

▶ *Interactive Skills CD:* Charting Procedures.

▶ *Dental Terminology, Third Edition:* Chapter 7, Examination and Prevention.

▶ *Delmar's Dental Assisting Exam Review:* Additional review material, test questions, and rationales provide practice for the DANB examination.

▶ *CourseMate:* Additional practice exercises that further reinforce Chapter 14 content can be found on the CourseMate Web site.

▶ *Dental Assisting Coloring Book:* Additional practice exercises that further reinforce Chapter 14 content.

▶ *Recommended minimum time to complete Chapter 14:* 5 to 6 hours, depending on depth of information the instructor wishes to cover.

LECTURE OUTLINE CORRELATED TO INSTRUCTOR PRESENTATIONS IN POWERPOINT

The presentations provided contain lecture notes. The notes can be viewed in PowerPoint when viewing the slides in either the normal or outline view. To print the slides with the notes: From your print box look for the "Print What" and change the drop-down to "Notes Pages." A new feature called "Dental Checks" has been interspersed throughout the presentations to keep the student engaged in the materials during the lecture. This feature contains a quick question followed by the answer to stimulate a brief discussion.

1. Dental Charts (Slide 2)

2. Numbering Systems (Slides 3 through 9)

    a. Universal/National System for Numbering

    b. Fédération Dentaire Internationale (FDI) System for Numbering

    c. Palmer System for Numbering

3. Cavity Classifications (Slides 11 through 17)

    a. Class I

    b. Class II

    c. Class III

    d. Class IV

    e. Class V

    f. Class VI

4. Abbreviations of Tooth Surfaces (Slides 19 through 22)

5. Basic Charting Terms (Slides 24 through 27)

6. Charting Color Indications and Symbols (Slide 28)

TEACHING STRATEGIES

1. Chapter contents are presented in the PowerPoint slides, which are found in the Electronic Classroom Manager to Accompany Delmar's *Dental Assisting*.

2. It is beneficial to have the students take a specific chart and chart each symbol on it. For instance, have the students start with tooth #1 to be removed. They can chart this on their own copy (which can later become a study guide) and label it. In this way, they can practice while also developing a reference.

3. Charting exercises are the best practice. The instructor can read aloud the charting for the students to complete on the computer or manually on a patient chart. When completed, the instructor can show the class a correctly completed chart. Students can then compare their own results with those of the instructor.

4. The instructor can proceed through a charting exercise or give the students a written copy and then take it back and question the students about what they have charted. An example is, "How many surfaces of decay are shown on this chart?" The students would have to count the notations that they made on their chart. Another example is, "What is the number of the tooth that needs root canal therapy?" The students would have to look at their chart and find the tooth that was charted for root canal therapy.

5. A quiz or a Web assignment can be required of the students to again review the material and broaden their knowledge base.

6. Have each student complete the two charting exercises in the textbook without looking at the answers.

7. Models can be made and painted in gold, silver, and cream colors to indicate restorations. Other findings can be written on a card. The students can chart the visual findings, followed by the written findings, and then be given the correct charting indications so that they can evaluate their performance. This can be done in a group as well.

CASE STUDY ANSWERS

Case Study 1

1. Tooth #9 has Class III mesial caries.

2. Ten teeth are restored, including the restoration with recurrent decay and the bridge abutments and pontic.

3. Tooth #20 is a pontic.

Case Study 2

1. Tooth #14 has an enamel sealant.

2. Tooth #73 is a primary tooth that is present in the patient's mouth.

3. Tooth #34 needs endodontic therapy.

TEXTBOOK REVIEW ANSWERS

Multiple Choice

1. d	2. c	3. b	4. c	5. a	6. c	7. d	8. b
9. a	10. d						

Critical Thinking

1. The five surfaces on an anterior tooth are mesial, distal, facial (labial), lingual, and incisal. The mesial, distal, and lingual are the same for a posterior tooth.

2. (Universal) MI, Class IV on teeth #8 and #9. (ISO) or (FDI) MI, Class IV on teeth #11 and #21. (Palmer) MI, Class IV on teeth.

3. It could be charted in red or blue, depending on the dentist's preference. See the textbook for more information.

Pharmacology

SPECIFIC INSTRUCTIONAL OBJECTIVES

1. Identify terms related to drugs, pharmacology, and medicines.

2. Identify the difference between drug brand names and generic names.

3. Identify the parts of a written prescription.

4. Identify the texts pertinent to pharmacology.

5. Give the English meanings of the Latin abbreviations used for prescriptions.

6. Specify the drug laws and who enforces them.

7. Identify the schedules for the Comprehensive Drug Abuse Prevention and Control Act of 1970.

8. Identify the routes through which drugs can be administered.

9. Demonstrate an understanding of the drugs used in dentistry and the ways in which they are used.

10. Summarize the uses and effects of nicotine, caffeine, alcohol, marijuana, and cocaine.

11. Summarize information about heroin, morphine, and codeine.

12. Supply information about amphetamines.

13. Demonstrate an understanding of hallucinogenic drugs such as LSD, PCP, and mescaline.

14. Demonstrate an understanding of barbiturates.

PREPARATORY

Personnel

Primary instructor who is knowledgeable about pharmacology and how it pertains to dental assisting. If instructor is not a dental assistant, a pharmacy tech or pharmacist can teach this content as long as it relates to the dental office.

Suggested Audiovisual and Resource Materials

▶ *Workbook:* Chapter 15.

▶ *Image Library:* Provides illustrations from Chapter 15 of the textbook that can be used via computer or as transparencies to provide visual support for classroom instruction.

▶ *Computerized Test Bank:* Provides additional test questions for Chapter 15 and related material on the DANB examination.

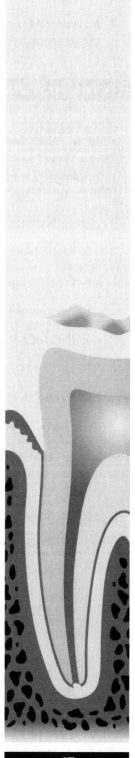

▶ *Practice Software:* Additional practice exercises that further reinforce Chapter 15 content can be found on the companion software disk.

▶ *Dental Terminology, Third Edition:* Chapter 8, Pain Management and Pharmacology.

▶ *Delmar's Dental Assisting Exam Review:* Additional review material, test questions, and rationales provide practice for the DANB examination.

▶ *CourseMate:* Additional practice exercises that further reinforce Chapter 15 content can be found on the CourseMate Web site.

▶ *Recommended minimum time to complete Chapter 15:* 3 to 4 hours, depending on depth of information the instructor wishes to cover.

LECTURE OUTLINE CORRELATED TO INSTRUCTOR PRESENTATIONS IN POWERPOINT

The presentations provided contain lecture notes. The notes can be viewed in PowerPoint when viewing the slides in either the normal or outline view. To print the slides with the notes: From your print box look for the "Print What" and change the drop-down to "Notes Pages." A new feature called "Dental Checks" has been interspersed throughout the presentations to keep the student engaged in the materials during the lecture. This feature contains a quick question followed by the answer to stimulate a brief discussion.

1. Drug Names (Slides 2 and 3)

    a. Brand Names

    b. Generic Names

2. Prescriptions (Slides 4 through 7)

    a. Parts of a Prescription

3. Drug Laws (Slides 9 through 13)

    a. Drug Schedule for the Comprehensive Abuse Prevention and Control Act of 1970

    b. Dental Assistants and the Law (Slide 15)

4. Drug Administration Routes (Slides 16 and 17)

    a. Oral

    b. Topical

    c. Inhalation

    d. Sublingual

    e. Rectal

    f. Intravenous

    g. Intramuscular

    h. Subcutaneous

    i. Intradermal

    j. Transdermal

5. Drugs (Slides 19 through 34)

    a. Analgesic

    b. Antibiotic

    c. Anticholinergic

    d. Anticoagulant

    e. Anticonvulsant

    f. Antidiabetic

    g. Antidepressant

    h. Antifungal

    i. Antihistamine

    j. Antihypertensive

    k. Anti-inflammatory

    l. Antilipemic

    m. Antithyroid

    n. Bronchodilator

    o. Contraceptive

    p. Decongestant

    q. Diuretic

    r. Hemostatic

    s. Hormone replacement

    t. MAOIs

    u. Nitrates

    v. Tranquilizer/anti-anxiety

6. Drugs Not Prescribed (Slides 36 through 45)

    a. Nicotine

    b. Caffeine

    c. Alcohol

    d. Marijuana

    e. Cocaine

    f. Narcotics

    g. Amphetamines

   h. Hallucinogens

   i. Barbiturates

 7. Herbal and Other Alternative Medications (Slide 47)

TEACHING STRATEGIES

1. Chapter contents are presented in the PowerPoint slides, which are found in the Instructor Resources to Accompany Delmar's *Dental Assisting*.

2. Numerous videos are available in school and public libraries on drugs and the effects they have on the body. Videos on herbal and other alternative medications are also available. These are a good tool to break up lecture content and encourage discussion.

3. Students could be placed in groups and asked to create a presentation on one of the drug groups listed in the textbook. The presentation can be tailored to pertain to dentistry and how such drugs would affect dental treatment.

4. Use a summary chart that includes pictures of drug types. A guest speaker from the local police department or a pharmacist may be available to address this topic.

5. Students can be assigned to look up a specific drug in the *Physician's Desk Reference* and hand in a report on what they learned, such as side effects, dosage, and so on.

CASE STUDY ANSWERS

1. The tobacco and the caffeine found in espresso, soft drinks, and chocolate act to speed up the body's metabolism.

2. These drugs are stimulants.

3. Due to drug interaction, this may be a problem, and it may change the intended result.

TEXTBOOK REVIEW ANSWERS

Multiple Choice

1. d 2. c 3. a 4. b 5. d 6. a 7. c 8. c

9. b 10. d

Critical Thinking

1. Patients may come to the dental office after taking an illegal drug, and, if the dental assistant has knowledge in this area, he or she can be better prepared to care for the patient, handle emergency situations, be alerted to the symptoms, and watch for drug interactions.

2. The side effects of tetracycline are nausea, vomiting, diarrhea, and possible rash. It is contraindicated in individuals with poor kidney function, children under 12, and pregnant women because it discolors developing teeth.

3. An anticholinergic drug, atropine, would reduce the heavy flow of saliva.

CHAPTER 16

Emergency Management

SPECIFIC INSTRUCTIONAL OBJECTIVES

1. Describe several emergency situations that may take place in the dental office. Explain how dental assistants can be prepared for these possibilities.

2. Describe the "CAB" approach to CPR and demonstrate the associated skills.

3. Define the terms and anatomy used in CPR delivery. Determine if the patient is unconscious and demonstrate knowledge of opening the airway and when and how to deliver chest compressions.

4. Identify several causes of airway obstructions in the dental office. Demonstrate the ability to open the airway and to perform the Heimlich maneuver.

5. Identify the causes, signs, and treatments for syncope, asthma, allergic reactions, anaphylactic reaction, hyperventilation, epilepsy, diabetes mellitus, hypoglycemia, angina pectoris, myocardial infarction, congestive heart failure, and stroke/cerebrovascular accident.

6. Identify several dental emergencies that a patient may have, such as abscessed tooth, alveolitis, avulsed tooth, broken prosthesis, soft tissue injury, broken tooth, and loose crown.

7. Gain an understanding of how a pulse oximeter, capnography, and electrocardiography work and how they are used in the dental office.

PREPARATORY

Primary instructor can be from the EMT area or a dental assisting instructor that has his or her BLS instructor card and a current BLS card. The instructor from the EMT area should be informed about the emergencies that occur in dental offices.

▶ *Workbook:* Chapter 16.

▶ *Image Library:* Provides illustrations from Chapter 16 of the textbook that can be used via computer or as transparencies to provide visual support for classroom instruction.

▶ *Computerized Test Bank:* Provides additional test questions for Chapter 16 and related material on the DANB examination.

▶ *Practice Software:* Additional practice exercises that further reinforce Chapter 16 content can be found on the companion software disk.

▶ *Dental Terminology, Third Edition:* Chapter 6, Emergency Care.

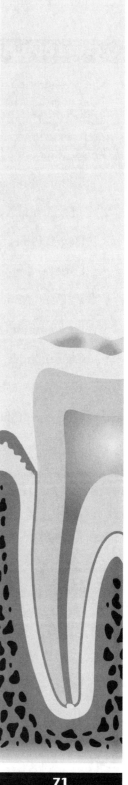

❱ ***Delmar's Dental Assisting Exam Review:*** Additional review material, test questions, and rationales provide practice for the DANB examination.

❱ ***CourseMate:*** Additional practice exercises that further reinforce Chapter 16 content can be found on the CourseMate Web site.

❱ ***Recommended minimum time to complete Chapter 16:*** 2 to 3 hours, depending on depth of information the instructor wishes to cover, plus 4 to 6 hours to complete the content and obtain a BLS card in adult and child CPR and choking prevention.

LECTURE OUTLINE CORRELATED TO INSTRUCTOR PRESENTATIONS IN POWERPOINT

The presentations provided contain lecture notes. The notes can be viewed in PowerPoint when viewing the slides in either the normal or outline view. To print the slides with the notes: From your print box look for the "Print What" and change the drop-down to "Notes Pages." A new feature called "Dental Checks" has been interspersed throughout the presentations to keep the student engaged in the materials during the lecture. This feature contains a quick question followed by the answer to stimulate a brief discussion.

1. Routine Preparedness for Dental Team Members (Slide 2)

2. The Dental Assistant's Role in Emergency Care (Slide 3)

3. Dental Office Emergency Kit (Slides 4 through 17)

4. Cardiopulmonary Resuscitation (Slides 19 and 20)

   a. The CAB of CPR

5. Foreign Body Airway Obstruction (Slides 21 through 25)

6. Causes, Signs, and Treatment of Emergencies (Slides 27 and 28)

   a. Syncope (Slides 29 through 33)

   b. Asthma (Slides 34 and 35)

   c. Orthostatic Hypotension (Slide 36)

   d. Allergic Reactions

   e. Anaphylactic Reaction (Slides 37 through 39)

   f. Hyperventilation (Slides 40 and 41)

   g. Epilepsy/Seizure Disorder (Slides 42 through 44)

   h. Diabetes Mellitus (Slides 45 through 49)

   i. Hypoglycemia (Slides 50 through 52)

   j. Cardiovascular Emergencies

   k. Angina Pectoris (Slide 53)

   l. Myocardial Infarction (Slides 54 and 55)

   m. Congestive Heart Failure (Slide 56)

   n. Stroke/Cerebrovascular Accident (Slide 57)

7. Dental Emergencies (Slide 58)

   a. Abscessed Tooth

   b. Alveolitis

   c. Avulsed Tooth

   d. Broken Prosthesis

   e. Soft Tissue Injury

   f. Broken Tooth

   g. Loose Permanent or Temporary Crown

8. Monitoring Patient's Health During Treatment (Slides 60 through 63)

   a. Pulse oximetry

   b. Capnography

   c. Electrocardiography

TEACHING STRATEGIES

1. Chapter contents are presented in the PowerPoint slides, which are found in the Instructor Resources to Accompany Delmar's *Dental Assisting*.

2. Numerous videos are available on emergencies. The American Heart Association has videos prepared for training to obtain a BLS card. The video is watched, the content is demonstrated, and then students practice the skills and perform them at a certain proficiency level. A video developed at the University of Kentucky shows several emergency situations, and leaves time for the students to decide what occurred and talk about the treatment for this emergency.

3. Students can role-play an emergency and have other students respond to this emergency.

4. Students can be organized into groups and asked to present a certain emergency situation and what should be done if it occurs in the dental office.

CASE STUDY ANSWERS

1. Thelma is probably experiencing a cerebrovascular accident (stroke).

2. The dental team should stop all dental treatment and remove any items from the patient's mouth. Position the patient so that the head is slightly elevated. Administer oxygen and monitor vital signs as emergency medical help is summoned. Provide CPR as needed.

3. Calming and reassuring the patient are important. Stress and apprehension may worsen the condition.

TEXTBOOK REVIEW ANSWERS

Multiple Choice

1. a   2. c   3. d   4. b   5. a   6. b   7. d   8. b

9. b   10. a

Critical Thinking

1. The dental team should stop dental treatment and remove items that may harm the patient. If the seizure is over in 5 minutes, place the patient in the recovery position and reassure him or her.

2. If the patient remains conscious, stop dental treatment and give the patient a sugar source, such as orange juice. If she or he becomes unconscious, terminate dental treatment, summon medical assistance, perform basic life support as needed, and, if necessary, administer an injection of glucagon or a sugar source such as cake icing gel placed in the buccal mucosa.

3. Arteriosclerosis is the condition, and it is commonly called hardening of the arteries.

Introduction to the Dental Office and Basic Chairside Assisting

SPECIFIC INSTRUCTIONAL OBJECTIVES

1. Describe the design of a dental office, explaining the purpose of each area.

2. Describe the equipment and function of the equipment in each area.

5. Describe the daily routine to open and close the dental office.

3. Explain basic concepts of chairside assisting.

6. Identify the activity zones and classifications of motions.

4. Describe the necessary steps to prepare the treatment room.

7. Explain the necessary steps to seat the patient for treatment.

8. Describe the ergonomics of the operator and the assistant at chairside.

9. Describe the necessary steps to dismiss the patient after treatment is finished.

10. Identify the special needs of certain patients.

PREPARATORY

Materials

Access to a reception/business area, dental treatment room, sterilization area, x-ray exposure and processing equipment, and dental laboratory. Include small equipment required in each of these areas. If you do not have access to all materials, you can use pictures, Web sites, and information from manufacturers and sales representatives.

Personnel

Primary instructor who is knowledgeable about the dental profession and understands the information the dental assistant needs to know to become familiar with all aspects of a dental office/clinic and to successfully function in a dental office. Instructor should be a Certified Dental Assistant.

The number of students in a class will determine the number of instructors needed for this topic because there are both lecture and clinical portions. In the clinical portion, the student will require hands-on instruction and learning activities that are better accomplished in smaller groups.

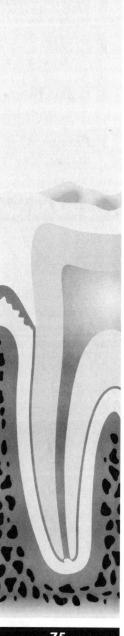

Suggested Audiovisual and Resource Materials

◗ *Workbook:* Chapter 17.

◗ *Delmar's Dental Assisting Video Series:* Appropriate content is available on Tape 1, *Chairside Assisting*. This includes seating and dismissing the patient.

◗ *Image Library:* Provides illustrations from Chapter 17 of the textbook that can be used via computer or as transparencies to provide visual support for classroom instruction.

◗ *Computerized Test Bank:* Provides additional test questions for Chapter 17 and related material on the DANB examination.

◗ *Practice Software:* Additional practice exercises that further reinforce Chapter 17 content can be found on the companion software disk.

◗ *Dental Terminology, Third Edition:* Chapter 4, Practice and Facility Setups.

◗ *Delmar's Dental Assisting Exam Review:* Additional review material, test questions, and rationales provide practice for the DANB examination.

◗ *CourseMate:* Additional practice exercises that further reinforce Chapter 17 content can be found on the CourseMate Web site.

◗ *Dental Assisting Coloring Book:* Additional practice exercises that further reinforce Chapter 17 content— see Chapter 6.

◗ *Recommended minimum time to complete Chapter 17:* 4 to 6 hours, depending on depth of information the instructor wishes to cover.

LECTURE OUTLINE CORRELATED TO INSTRUCTOR PRESENTATIONS IN POWERPOINT

The presentations provided contain lecture notes. The notes can be viewed in PowerPoint when viewing the slides in either the normal or outline view. To print the slides with the notes: From your print box look for the "Print What" and change the drop-down to "Notes Pages." A new feature called "Dental Checks" has been interspersed throughout the presentations to keep the student engaged in the materials during the lecture. This feature contains a quick question followed by the answer to stimulate a brief discussion.

1. Dental Office Design (Slides 2 and 3)

   a. Reception Room

   b. Reception Desk and Business Office

   c. Sterilizing Area

   d. Dental Office Laboratory

   e. X-Ray Processing Room

   f. Radiography Room

   g. Optional Rooms in the Dental Office

2. Treatment Rooms and Dental Equipment (Slides 4 through 7)

 a. The Dental Chair

 b. The Dental Unit

  i. Rear, side, and front delivery

  ii. Air-water syringe

  iii. Dental handpiece

  iv. Ultrasonic scaler

  v. Saliva ejector

  vi. High-volume evacuator

 c. Dental Stools

 d. Operating Light

 e. Cabinetry

 f. Sink

 g. Dental X-Ray Unit

 h. Small Equipment Found in the Treatment Room

  i. X-ray viewbox

  ii. Curing light

  iii. Radiometer

  iv. Amalgamator

  v. Communication system

  vi. Computer equipment

 i. Dental Air Compressor and Central Vacuum System

3. Routine Office Care (Slide 9)

 a. Operating and Closing the Dental Office

4. Concepts of Dental Assisting (Slide 10)

5. Activity Zones (Slide 11)

 a. Classifications of Motion (Slide 12)

6. Preparing the Treatment Room (Slide 14)

7. Seating the Dental Patient (Slide 15)

 a. Greet and Escort the Patient

 b. Seat and Prepare the Patient

8. Ergonomics for the Operator and the Assistant (Slides 16 through 19)

   a. Ergonomics for the Operator

   b. Ergonomics for the Assistant

9. Dismissing the Patient (Slide 20)

10. Patients with Special Needs (Slide 21)

   a. Child Patients

   b. Senior Patients

   c. Pregnant Patients

   d. Hearing-Impaired or Blind Patients

   e. Patients with Wheelchairs or Walkers

   f. Non-English-Speaking Patients

TEACHING STRATEGIES

1. Chapter contents are presented in the PowerPoint slides, which are found in the Instructor Resources to Accompany Delmar's *Dental Assisting*.

2. Much of the content in this chapter must be remembered by the student and then applied in the clinic setting.

3. The student should become familiar with the common areas found in most dental offices/clinics. Have the students discuss their own personal dental experiences by asking them to describe the office and what they saw in these areas. After the discussion, the students should have a general idea and then you can fill in the details of the equipment and materials found in each area.

4. Bring in a sales representative to show various types of equipment and materials found in the dental office/clinic. Use the Web as a learning tool. Activity: Divide the office into sections, and assign each student an area or piece of equipment that he or she needs to research and report back to the class.

5. Demonstrate to the class how to prepare for a patient, seat a patient, and dismiss a patient, including all of the items found in Chapter 17 of the workbook.

6. Discuss the ergonomic concepts of the dentist and dental assistant, and demonstrate the correct positions when working on a patient.

CASE STUDY ANSWERS

1. Mrs. Rose might feel light-headed after being reclined for a period of time.

2. The assistant can seat Mrs. Rose upright and allow her to remain so for a few minutes before proceeding to the reception room.

3. If time allows during the procedure, the assistant can elevate Mrs. Rose's head.

TEXTBOOK REVIEW ANSWERS

Multiple Choice

1. c   2. b   3. b   4. b   5. b   6. c   7. a   8. c

9. d   10. b

Critical Thinking

1. The office should be clean and orderly, with current magazines; bright; accessible; and maintained at a comfortable climate. Dental information should be available for patients of all ages. Someone should greet the patients as they enter the office and as they leave.

2. Good visibility of the patient's mouth; easy access to all areas of the patient's mouth; easy access to dental equipment, instruments, and materials; safety and comfort for the patient, operator, and assistant.

3. Keep the appointments short, allow for breaks, seat the patient in a more upright position, and readjust the chair occasionally.

Basic Chairside Instruments and Tray Systems

SPECIFIC INSTRUCTIONAL OBJECTIVES

1. Identify the parts of an instrument.

2. Describe how instruments are identified.

3. Identify the categories and functions of dental burs.

4. Describe the types and functions of abrasives.

5. Explain various handpieces and attachments.

6. Describe types of tray systems and color-coding systems.

PREPARATORY

Materials

Various dental hand instruments; slow-speed and high-speed dental handpieces; various burs, discs, and stones; high-volume evacuator; saliva ejector; cotton rolls; and gauze. In addition, various trays, tubs, tray mats, tray systems, and color-coding systems should be available.

Personnel

Primary instructor who is knowledgeable about the dental profession and understands the information the dental assistant must know to become familiar with basic and restorative instruments; dental handpieces; burs, discs, and stones; and various tray systems and color-coding systems.

The number of students in a class will determine the number of instructors needed for this chapter because there are both lecture and clinical portions. In the clinical portion, the student requires hands-on instruction and learning activities that are better accomplished in smaller groups. The instructor should be a Certifed Dental Assistant.

Suggested Audiovisual and Resource Materials

▶ *Workbook:* Chapter 18.

▶ *Image Library:* Provides illustrations from Chapter 18 of the textbook that can be used via computer or as transparencies to provide visual support for classroom instruction.

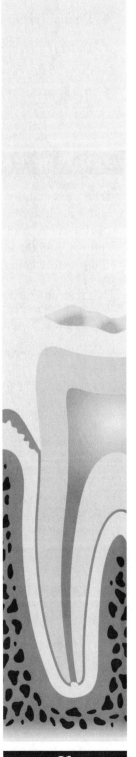

▶ *Computerized Test Bank:* Provides additional test questions for Chapter 18 and related material on the DANB examination.

▶ *Practice Software:* Additional practice exercises that further reinforce Chapter 18 content can be found on the companion software disk.

▶ *CourseMate:* Additional practice exercises that further reinforce Chapter 18 content can be found on the CourseMate Web site.

▶ *Dental Assisting Instrument Guide:* For review of instrumentation covered in Chapter 18.

▶ *Dental Terminology, Third Edition:* Chapter 4, Practice and Facility Setups.

▶ *Delmar's Dental Assisting Exam Review:* Additional review material, test questions, and rationales provide practice for the DANB examination.

▶ *Recommended minimum time to complete Chapter 18:* 4 to 6 hours, depending on depth of information the instructor wishes to cover and the skill level required by students.

LECTURE OUTLINE CORRELATED TO INSTRUCTOR PRESENTATIONS IN POWERPOINT

The presentations provided contain lecture notes. The notes can be viewed in PowerPoint when viewing the slides in either the normal or outline view. To print the slides with the notes: From your print box look for the "Print What" and change the drop-down to "Notes Pages." A new feature called "Dental Checks" has been interspersed throughout the presentations to keep the student engaged in the materials during the lecture. This feature contains a quick question followed by the answer to stimulate a brief discussion.

1. Instruments for Basic Chairside Procedures

    a. Basic Structural Parts of Dental Hand Instruments (Slide 2)

        i. Working end

        ii. Handle

        iii. Shank

    b. Basic Classification of Dental Instruments (Slides 3 through 6)

        i. Number of working ends

        ii. Function

        iii. Manufacturer's number

        iv. Black's formula

    c. Cutting Instruments (Slides 8 through 13)

        i. Chisel

        ii. Hatchet

        iii. Hoe

        iv. Gingival margin trimmer

      v. Angle former

      vi. Excavator

    d. Noncutting Instruments (Slides 15 through 21)

      i. Basic: mouth mirror, explorer, cotton pliers, periodontal probe

      ii. Plastic filling instrument

      iii. Composite instrument

      iv. Amalgam carrier

      v. Amalgam condenser

      vi. Carver

      vii. Burnisher

      viii. File

      ix. Finishing knife

    e. Miscellaneous Instruments (Slide 22)

      i. Spatula

      ii. Articulating forcep

      iii. Scissor

    f. Instrument Care, Maintenance, and Sterilization (Slide 23)

2. Dental Rotary Instruments (Slides 25 and 26)

    a. Parts of the Bur

      i. Shank

      ii. Neck

      iii. Head

    b. Cutting Burs

    c. Diamond Burs

    d. Finishing Burs

    e. Surgical Burs

    f. Laboratory Burs

    g. Fissurotomy Burs

3. Abrasives (Slides 27 through 30)

    a. Mandrels

    b. Discs

    c. Stones

    d. Rubber Wheels

    e. Rubber Points

    f. Sterilization, Maintenance, and Storage

4. Dental Handpieces (Slides 32 through 35)

    a. Parts of the Dental Handpiece

    b. High-Speed Handpiece

    c. Low-Speed Handpiece

    d. Electric Handpiece

    e. Maintenance and Sterilization of Dental Handpieces (Slide 35)

5. Air Abrasion Unit (Slide 36)

6. Microetcher (Slide 36)

7. Tray Systems (Slide 37)

    a. Positioning on Trays

    b. Cassette System for Instruments

    c. Color-Coding Systems (Slides 38 and 39)

TEACHING STRATEGIES

1. Chapter contents are presented in the PowerPoint slides, which are found in the Instructor Resources to Accompany Delmar's *Dental Assisting*.

2. Much of the content in this chapter must be remembered by the student and applied in the clinic setting.

3. Students should read the chapter and after the lecture they should have hands-on time to learn the instruments, handpieces, burs, discs, and stones. A variety of items should be available so that they can learn the different shapes and how to handle the instruments. Have the students use *Delmar's Dental Assisting Instrument Guide* to assist their learning the instruments, handpieces, burs, and so on.

4. Have the students identify each instrument and its function, which tray setup it would be used in, and where in the sequence of the procedure it is used.

5. Have a variety of tray systems and color-coding systems for the student to examine and have them explain how color-coding systems work in the dental office.

CASE STUDY ANSWERS

1. Whether the color coding is going to indicate procedures, treatment rooms, individual operators, and/or number of sets of instruments.

2. One example is a two-color tray setup; blue, for instance, indicates amalgam, and another color would indicate which of four amalgam tray setups. Another example is diagonal color coding of instruments to indicate sequence of use. A third example in a two-operator office is as follows: blue indicates procedure; diagonal yellow indicates sequence and set; and a third color, red, identifies the operator. (The other operator would be identified via green as the third color.)

3. Color coding allows easy identification of instruments by procedures, treatment room, and operators, which helps the dental assistant to keep the instruments separate for easier preparation during sterilization, tray setups, and use.

TEXTBOOK REVIEW ANSWERS

Multiple Choice

1. b   2. b   3. d   4. a   5. c   6. d   7. a   8. c

9. b   10. b

Critical Thinking

1. The bur number identifies the shape, size, and variation of the bur.

2. The dental assistant would select a low-speed handpiece, and a right-angle (prophy) attachment would be required.

3. The basic hand instruments necessary for an amalgam restoration procedure include: basic setup, spoon excavator, (possibly) manual cutting instruments, amalgam carrier, amalgam condenser, carvers, and articulating forceps and paper.

4. First color-code each dentist or hygienist with a different color—requires four different colors, one for each operator. Second color-code each set of instruments—requires two colors. There are two ways to indicate the sequence/order the instruments need to be placed on the tray: One way is to place the second color diagonally on the instruments. The second way is to add another color to show the sequence/order.

CHAPTER 19

Instrument Transfer and Maintaining the Operating Field

SPECIFIC INSTRUCTIONAL OBJECTIVES

1. Describe the transfer zone.

2. Define a fulcrum and tactile sensation.

3. Describe the grasps, positions, and transfer of instruments for a procedure.

4. List the eight rules for instrument transfer.

5. Understand instrument transfer modification.

6. Describe and demonstrate how to maintain the oral cavity.

7. Explain the equipment used in the treatment of the oral cavity.

8. Describe techniques for moisture control and isolation.

9. Explain techniques for dental assistants performing expanded functions.

PREPARATORY

Materials

Various dental hand instruments, slow-speed and high-speed dental handpiece, high-volume evacuator, saliva ejector, cotton rolls, gauze, mannequin, dental chair, dental unit, dentist's stool, and dental assistant's stool.

Personnel

Primary instructor who is knowledgeable about the dental profession and understands the information the dental assistant needs to know to become skilled at chairside assisting, including instrument transfer and maintaining the operation field.

Because this topic includes both lecture and clinical portions, the number of students in a class will determine the number of instructors. In the clinical portion, the student will require hands-on instruction and learning activities that are better accomplished in smaller groups. The instructor should be a Certified Dental Assistant.

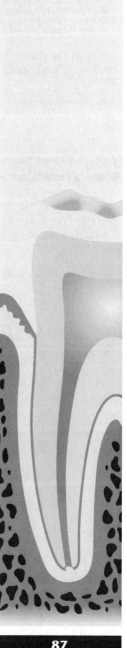

Suggested Audiovisual and Resource Materials

❱ *Workbook:* Chapter 19.

❱ *Delmar's Dental Assisting Video Series:* Appropriate content is available on Tape 1, *Chairside Assisting.* This includes one-handed instrument transfer techniques and placement of the HVE tip.

❱ *Image Library:* Provides illustrations from Chapter 19 of the textbook that can be used via computer or as transparencies to provide visual support for classroom instruction.

❱ *Computerized Test Bank:* Provides additional test questions for Chapter 19 and related material on the DANB examination.

❱ *Practice Software:* Additional practice exercises that further reinforce Chapter 19 content can be found on the companion software disk.

❱ *Dental Terminology, Third Edition:* Chapter 4, Practice and Facility Setups.

❱ *Delmar's Dental Assisting Exam Review:* Additional review material, test questions, and rationales provide practice for the DANB examination.

❱ *CourseMate:* Additional practice exercises that further reinforce Chapter 19 content can be found on the CourseMate Web site.

❱ *Recommended minimum time to complete Chapter 19:* 4 to 6 hours, depending on depth of information the instructor wishes to cover and the skill level required by students.

LECTURE OUTLINE CORRELATED TO INSTRUCTOR PRESENTATIONS IN POWERPOINT

The presentations provided contain lecture notes. The notes can be viewed in PowerPoint when viewing the slides in either the normal or outline view. To print the slides with the notes: From your print box look for the "Print What" and change the drop-down to "Notes Pages." A new feature called "Dental Checks" has been interspersed throughout the presentations to keep the student engaged in the materials during the lecture. This feature contains a quick question followed by the answer to stimulate a brief discussion.

1. Instrument Transfer (Slides 2 through 12)

    a. Transfer Hand

    b. Instrument Grasps

        i. Pen grasp

        ii. Modified pen grasp

        iii. Palm grasp

        iv. Palm-thumb grasp

        v. Reverse palm-thumb grasp

    c. Instrument Transfer Methods

        i. One handed

        ii. Two handed

　　d. Instrument Transfer Modifications (Slides 14 through 18)

　　　　i. Mirror and explorer transfer

　　　　ii. Cotton pliers transfer

　　　　iii. Scissors transfer

　　　　iv. Dental handpieces

　　　　v. Air-water syringe transfer

　　　　vi. Miscellaneous

2. Maintaining the Operating Field (Slides 19 through 28)

　　a. Lighting

　　b. The Evacuation System

　　　　i. Placements

　　　　ii. Grasps

　　　　iii. Guidelines

　　c. Saliva Ejector

　　d. The Air-Water Syringe

　　e. Retraction of Tissues

　　　　i. Mouth mirror

　　　　ii. Rubber dam

　　　　iii. Evacuator tip

　　　　iv. Cotton rolls or gauze

　　　　v. Tissue retractors

　　　　vi. Mouth props

　　　　vii. Isolite system

3. Techniques for Moisture Control and Isolation (Slides 29 and 30)

　　a. Cotton Rolls

　　b. Dry Angles

4. Expanded Functions (Slide 31)

TEACHING STRATEGIES

1. Chapter contents are presented in the PowerPoint slides, which are found in the Instructor Resources to Accompany Delmar's *Dental Assisting*.

2. Much of the content in this chapter must be remembered by the student and applied in the clinic setting. A study guide may assist in the student's retention of this material.

3. Have the students discuss personal dental experiences by having them describe the treatment they received during dental visits, as well as what the dental assistant was doing to assist the dentist.

4. Show the video on instrument transfer and oral evacuation, and then discuss the clinical aspects they should be aware of during chairside assisting.

5. Demonstrate to the class how to pass and receive dental instruments and how to evacuate the various quadrants. Have the students practice these skills on a mannequin until you feel comfortable with their skill level. They can then practice on student partners to gain confidence and effectiveness. Have the students follow the steps in the procedures found in Chapter 19 of the workbook.

6. Discuss with the class the importance of these basic chairside skills, how they are used with every patient, and how the students can enhance the dentist and the procedure by being the best dental assistants they can be.

CASE STUDY ANSWERS

1. Kaitlin can arrange the instruments and miscellaneous items on the tray in the sequence of the procedure. Have the patient ready, the light in position, and the handpieces and air-water syringe prepared and positioned.

2. Review the eight basic rules for instrument transfer and how to do the one-handed and two-handed instrument transfer.

3. The assistant is responsible for keeping the dentist's vision and access clear by making sure that the fluids are removed from the mouth and that the patient does not swallow or aspirate the fluids. The assistant also adjusts the dental light when necessary and keeps an eye on the patient.

TEXTBOOK REVIEW ANSWERS

Multiple Choice

1. a   2. a   3. d   4. d   5. d   6. a   7. b   8. b

9. d   10. b

Critical Thinking

1. Routine flushing of the system with water and chemical solutions helps to reduce the risk. This could be done after each patient, at the end of the day, and/or at the end of the week.

2. Review information on techniques for moisture control and isolation. Review information on salivary glands and ducts in Chapter 7, Head and Neck Anatomy.

3. The dentist would use a fulcrum to steady his or her hand when working with a dental instrument to ensure control. The dentist would select a stable surface such as the teeth or the gingival tissues. A 2 × 2 gauze is often used on the teeth and tissues to secure the fulcrum and prevent slipping.

Anesthesia and Sedation

SPECIFIC INSTRUCTIONAL OBJECTIVES

1. Describe the methods used to manage the pain and anxiety associated with dental procedures.

2. Explain various topical anesthetics and their placements.

3. Describe types of local anesthetics.

4. Identify the injection sites for the maxillary and mandibular arches.

5. Describe the equipment and materials needed to administer local anesthetic.

6. List the steps for preparing for the administration of local anesthetic.

7. Identify supplemental techniques to administer anesthetics.

8. Discuss the role of nitrous oxide in the care of the dental patient.

9. Demonstrate the ability to assist in the administration of nitrous oxide.

PREPARATORY

Personnel

Primary instructor who is knowledgeable about the dental profession and understands the information the dental assistant needs to know to become familiar with basic anesthesia and sedation administered in the dental office. This instructor should be a Certified Dental Assistant.

The number of students in a class will determine the number of instructors needed for this chapter because there are both lecture and clinical portions. In the clinical portion, the student requires hands-on instruction and learning activities that are better accomplished in smaller groups.

Suggested Audiovisual and Resource Materials

▶ *Workbook:* Chapter 20.

▶ *Image Library:* Provides illustrations from Chapter 20 of the textbook that can be used via computer or as transparencies to provide visual support for classroom instruction.

▶ *Computerized Test Bank:* Provides additional test questions for Chapter 20 and related material on the DANB examination.

▶ *Practice Software:* Additional practice exercises that further reinforce Chapter 20 content can be found on the companion software disk.

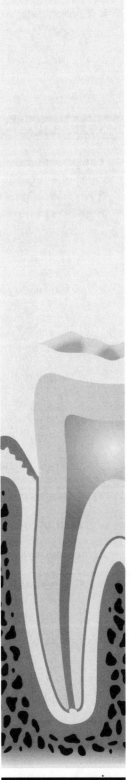

▶ *Interactive Skills CD:* Basic Operative Setups: Anesthetic.

▶ *Dental Terminology, Third Edition:* Chapter 8, Pharmacology.

▶ *Dental Assisting Instrument Guide:* Review of instrumentation discussed in Chapter 20.

▶ *Delmar's Dental Assisting Exam Review:* Additional review material, test questions, and rationales provide practice for the DANB examination.

▶ *CourseMate:* Additional practice exercises that further reinforce Chapter 20 content can be found on the CourseMate Web site.

▶ *Recommended minimum time to complete Chapter 20:* 4 to 6 hours, depending on the depth of information the instructor wishes to cover and the skill level required by students.

LECTURE OUTLINE CORRELATED TO INSTRUCTOR PRESENTATIONS IN POWERPOINT

The presentations provided contain lecture notes. The notes can be viewed in PowerPoint when viewing the slides in either the normal or outline view. To print the slides with the notes: From your print box look for the "Print What" and change the drop-down to "Notes Pages." A new feature called "Dental Checks" has been interspersed throughout the presentations to keep the student engaged in the materials during the lecture. This feature contains a quick question followed by the answer to stimulate a brief discussion.

1. Anesthetics and Sedation (Slide 2)

   a. Conscious Sedation (Slide 3)

   b. Intravenous Conscious Sedation (IV Sedation) (Slide 4)

   c. Oral Sedation (Slide 5)

   d. Inhalation Sedation (Slide 6)

   e. Intramuscular Sedation (Slide 7)

   f. General Anesthesia (Slide 8)

   g. Topical Anesthesia (Slide 9)

   h. Local Anesthesia (Slide 10)

2. Topical Anesthetics (Slides 11 and 12)

3. Local Anesthetics (Slides 13 and 14)

   a. Local Anesthetic Agents

   b. Vasoconstrictors

   c. Possible Complications of Local Anesthetics

   d. Types of Injections (Slides 16 through 20)

      i. Local infiltration

      ii. Field block

      iii. Nerve block

4. Injection Sites (Slides 21 and 22)

   a. Maxillary

   b. Mandibular

5. Anesthetics, Syringes, and Needles (Slides 24 through 33)

   a. Syringe

   b. Needle

   c. Anesthetic Cartridge

6. Supplemental Anesthetic Techniques

   a. Intraosseous Anesthesia (Slide 35)

   b. Periodontal Ligament Injection (Slides 36 and 37)

   c. Intrapulpal Injection (Slide 38)

   d. Electronic Anesthesia (Slide 39)

   e. Computer-Controlled Local Anesthesia Delivery System (Slide 40)

7. Nitrous Oxide Sedation (Slides 41 and 42)

   a. Safety and Precautions

   b. Indications for Use of Nitrous Oxide Sedation

   c. Contraindications for Use of Nitrous Oxide Sedation

   d. Equipment

TEACHING STRATEGIES

1. Chapter contents are presented in the PowerPoint slides, which are found in the Instructor Resources to Accompany Delmar's *Dental Assisting*.

2. The student must remember much of this chapter's content. A study guide in which the student must look up information and write it out is one way to help reinforce memory.

3. Students should read the chapter, and after the lecture proceed to hands-on practice to learn how to prepare, load, pass, and receive the anesthetic syringe.

4. Show the *Delmar's Dental Assisting* video on preparing, loading, passing, and receiving the anesthetic syringe.

5. In class, provide a needle for each student to examine and learn how to open. Distribute an anesthetic carpule for each student to examine, and review the information that is found on the mylar sheath that covers the carpule.

6. Provide students with a diagram to mark the sites where the topical anesthetic is placed and the local injection is given. Then have the students shade in the area that is affected by each injection. This is a good visual aid in learning injection sites since dental assistants in many states are allowed to place the topical anesthetic.

7. In the lab/clinic, have the students point out the injection sites on each other, while practicing placement of topical anesthetic.

8. Demonstrate how to prepare, load, pass, and receive the anesthetic syringe.

9. Invite a dentist to demonstrate nitrous oxide on each student in the clinical setting or visit a dental office for this purpose. Each student will understand how patients are affected by nitrous oxide after experiencing it themselves.

CASE STUDY ANSWERS

1. It is likely that no considerations in the patient's medical history would predict this reaction.

2. Overdose, or excessive anesthetic solution, is a possibility, as is an allergic reaction (which may or may not depend on dosage). Chuck is experiencing a toxic reaction to topical anesthetic.

3. The dental assistant should be on the alert for apprehensiveness in the patient.

TEXTBOOK REVIEW ANSWERS

Multiple Choice

1. b   2. a   3. b   4. b   5. b   6. b   7. d   8. d

9. c   10. d

Critical Thinking

1. The anesthetic solution with a vasoconstrictor, usually epinephrine, would be selected to provide a longer lasting pain control and promote less bleeding for the patient. The vasoconstrictor acts to constrict the blood vessels around the injection site and to reduce blood flow in this area, thus slowing the absorption of the anesthetic into the blood stream.

2. Type of anesthetic, percent of solution, number of cartridges administered, and any reaction the patient experienced should be noted.

3. Patients who would benefit the most are those who are nervous and apprehensive about dental treatment. Patients who have gag reflex sensitivity, cannot breathe through their noses, have heart conditions, and/or require long appointments would also benefit.

4. The patient is most likely having a toxic reaction to the anesthetic solution. The dental assistant should notify the dentist immediately and stay with the patient. Also note on the patient's chart that they had a reaction to the anesthetic solution and list the brand name, type, and the percentage of anesthetic and vasoconstrictor in the solution.

CHAPTER 21

Introduction to Dental Radiography and Equipment

SPECIFIC INSTRUCTIONAL OBJECTIVES

1. Explain the history of radiation and the use of the Hittorf-Crookes and Coolidge tubes.

2. List the properties of radiation and explain the biological effects of radiation exposure.

3. Identify the components of a dental x-ray unit and explain the function of each component.

4. Describe safety precautions when using radiation.

5. Explain how an x-ray is produced.

6. Describe the composition, sizes, types, and storage of dental x-ray film.

PREPARATORY

Personnel

Dental assisting instructors can teach the introduction to dental radiography class. They should have the radiology certification from DANB.

Suggested Audiovisual and Resource Materials

▶ *Workbook:* Chapter 21.

▶ *Image Library:* Provides illustrations from Chapter 21 of the textbook that can be used via computer or as transparencies to provide visual support for classroom instruction.

▶ *Computerized Test Bank:* Provides additional test questions for Chapter 21 and related material on the DANB examination.

▶ *Practice Software:* Additional practice exercises that further reinforce Chapter 21 content can be found on the companion software disk.

▶ *Interactive Skills CD:* Radiographs.

▶ *Dental Terminology, Third Edition:* Chapter 9, Radiography.

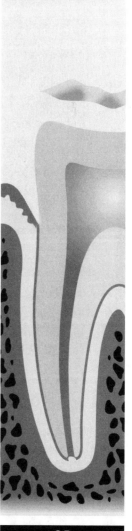

▶ *Dental Assisting Coloring Book:* Exercises for additional practice on topics presented in Chapter 21.

▶ *Delmar's Dental Assisting Exam Review:* Additional review material, test questions, and rationales provide practice for the DANB examination.

▶ *CourseMate:* Additional practice exercises that further reinforce Chapter 21 content can be found on the CourseMate Web site.

▶ *Recommended minimum time to complete Chapter 21:* 5 to 6 hours, depending on depth of information the instructor wishes to cover, plus additional hours in the dental laboratory to identify the equipment and demonstrate usage.

LECTURE OUTLINE CORRELATED TO INSTRUCTOR PRESENTATIONS IN POWERPOINT

The presentations provided contain lecture notes. The notes can be viewed in PowerPoint when viewing the slides in either the normal or outline view. To print the slides with the notes; from your print box look for the "Print What" and change the drop-down to "Notes Pages." A new feature called "Dental Checks" has been interspersed throughout the presentations to keep the student engaged in the materials during the lecture. This feature contains a quick question followed by the answer to stimulate a brief discussion.

1. Discovery of X-Rays (Slides 2 through 5)

   a. Roentgen

   b. Hittorf-Crookes

   c. Walkoff

   d. Kells

   e. Rollins

   f. Coolidge

   g. Victor X-Ray Corporation

   h. Rober and Cieszyski

   i. McCormack

   j. Fitzgerald and Updegrave

   k. Paatero

   l. Morris

   m. Digital Radiography

2. Radiation Physics and Biology (Slides 7 through 14)

   a. The Structure of an Atom and Ionization

   b. Radiation Types

   c. Radiation Units of Measurement

3. Biological Effects of Radiation (Slides 15 and 16)

   a. Somatic and Genetic Effects of Radiation

   b. Radiosensitive Cells

   c. Occupational Exposure

   d. Daily Radiation Exposure

   e. Accumulation of Radiation

4. Components of the Dental X-Ray Unit (Slides 18 and 19)

   a. Control Panel

   b. Arm Assembly and Tubehead

5. Safety and Precautions (Slide 20)

   a. Manufacturer's Responsibilities

   b. Dentist's Responsibilities

   c. Dental Assistant's Responsibilities

   d. Patient's Responsibilities

   e. Additional Notes on Reducing Radiation Exposure

6. Radiation Production (Slides 22 and 23)

7. Dental X-Ray Film (Slide 24)

   a. Composition of Dental X-Ray Film

   b. Film Speed

   c. Film Sizes

   d. Dental Film Packet

   e. Dental Film Storage

TEACHING STRATEGIES

1. Chapter contents are presented in the PowerPoint slides, which are found in the Instructor Resources to Accompany Delmar's *Dental Assisting*.

2. The student must remember much of this chapter's content. A study guide in which the student must look up information and write it out is one way to reinforce memory.

3. The radiation health and safety representative for the local area is often available to talk with students. Bring him or her in as a guest speaker to talk about the effects of radiation. Many times the speaker will bring equipment that measures radiation, and students can watch a demonstration about how radiation works. The students will gain an understanding about distance from the source, primary beam, and how KVP and MA affect the ray.

4. Students can label the unit and components to help in understanding.

5. Several movies about radiation are available that can be purchased from Kodak. One of the best ones for introducing radiography is *How Does Radiation Work?*

6. Allowing each student to open a film packet and examine the parts as the instructor discusses these elements is helpful. Providing students with various film sizes during demonstration is also useful. Refer students to Figures 21-14 and 21-15 in the textbook.

CASE STUDY ANSWERS

1. The redness is called erythema.

2. Dr. Scott should discontinue use of this technique.

3. If she continues using the technique, she may first lose her hand and later her life.

4. Dr. Scott could very likely lose her hand due to this procedure.

5. With unprotected continued radiation exposure, Dr. Scott could lose her life.

TEXTBOOK REVIEW ANSWERS

Multiple Choice

1. d   2. c   3. b   4. d   5. c   6. d   7. d   8. a

9. d   10. b

Critical Thinking

1. It is not sound thinking to turn down the kilovoltage. The kilovoltage speed allows the radiation to go through the tissues. To ensure that the patient receives minimal radiation a lead apron with thyroid collar should be used. The dental assistant should also use F-speed film with a rectangular PID to cut down the radiation exposure. Only necessary radiographs that are prescribed by the dentist should be exposed. The dental assistant should take care in taking the exposures so they will not need to be retaken.

2. Initially, radiographs should not be taken until the problem is solved. The dental assistant should be asked if the badge was worn outside of the office or if the badge was left inside the exposure room. It would be beneficial to compare this badge to others used in the same area. The high readings could have occurred due to taking the x-ray badge outside of the office or leaving it in a car or a window at home where it could have received exposure to the sun's rays.

3. The period between direct exposure and the development of biological effects or symptoms is called the latent period. Therefore the friend may come in from the sun exposure and not have the symptoms occur until several hours after the initial exposure. Yes, the skin of individuals who had high exposure to the sun will age at an increased rate.

Production and Evaluation of Dental Radiographs

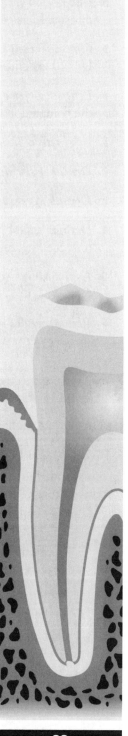

SPECIFIC INSTRUCTIONAL OBJECTIVES

1. Describe a diagnostic-quality x-ray.

2. Identify the means of producing quality radiographs.

3. List the types of film exposures.

4. Explain the bisecting principle and technique.

5. Explain the paralleling principle and techniques including a full-mouth radiographic survey and bite-wing series.

6. Describe special radiographs on various patients, including occlusal, pediatric, edentulous, and endodontic radiographs, and special needs/compromised patients.

7. Describe manual film-processing equipment and technique.

8. List and explain the composition of processing solutions.

9. Describe automatic processing equipment and explain the technique.

10. Explain and demonstrate how to mount dental x-rays.

11. List common radiographic errors that occur during exposure and processing of x-ray films.

12. Explain how to duplicate dental radiographs.

13. Describe the storage of final radiographs and legal implications concerning dental radiographs.

14. List standardized procedures and state policies that dental offices follow to ensure quality radiographs.

PREPARATORY

Personnel

Primary instructor who is knowledgeable about the dental profession and understands the information that the dental assistant needs to know to become familiar with producing and evaluating dental radiographs. This instructor should be a Certified Dental Assistant with the radiology certificate if required by his or her state Dental Practice Act.

The number of students in a class will determine the number of instructors needed for this chapter because there are both lecture and clinical portions. In the clinical portion, the student requires hands-on instruction and learning activities that are better accomplished in smaller groups.

Suggested Audiovisual and Resource Materials

▶ *Workbook:* Chapter 22.

▶ *Delmar's Dental Assisting Video Series:* Appropriate content is available on Tape 2, *Dental Radiography.* This includes infection control as well as exposing, processing, and mounting radiographs.

▶ *Image Library:* Provides illustrations from Chapter 22 of the textbook that can be used via computer or as transparencies to provide visual support for classroom instruction.

▶ *Computerized Test Bank:* Provides additional test questions for Chapter 22 and related material on the DANB examination.

▶ *Practice Software:* Additional practice exercises that further reinforce Chapter 22 content can be found on the companion software disk.

▶ *Interactive Skills CD:* Radiographs.

▶ *Dental Assisting Coloring Book:* Additional practice activities related to the content discussed in Chapter 22.

▶ *Dental Terminology, Third Edition:* Chapter 9, Radiography.

▶ *Delmar's Dental Assisting Exam Review:* Additional review material, test questions, and rationales provide practice for the DANB examination.

▶ *CourseMate:* Additional practice exercises that further reinforce Chapter 22 content can be found on the CourseMate Web site.

▶ *Recommended minimum time to complete Chapter 22:* 4 to 6 hours, depending on depth of information the instructor wishes to cover and the skill level required by students.

LECTURE OUTLINE CORRELATED TO INSTRUCTOR PRESENTATIONS IN POWERPOINT

The presentations provided contain lecture notes. The notes can be viewed in PowerPoint when viewing the slides in either the normal or outline view. To print the slides with the notes: From your print box look for the "Print What" and change the drop-down to "Notes Pages." A new feature called "Dental Checks" has been interspersed throughout the presentations to keep the student engaged in the materials during the lecture. This feature contains a quick question followed by the answer to stimulate a brief discussion.

1. Producing Quality Radiographs (Slide 2)

    a. Preparing for X-Ray Exposure

    b. During Film Exposure

    c. Patient Exposure

    d. After the Films Are Exposed

2. Types of Film Exposures (Slide 3)

   a. Periapical

   b. Bite-wing

   c. Occlusal

3. Intraoral Techniques for Film Exposures (Slides 9 through 11)

4. Bisecting Technique

   a. Principles

   b. Disadvantages

5. Full-Mouth Radiographic Survey

6. Bite-Wing Series

   a. Positioning for Maxillary Arch (Slides 10 through 13)

   b. Positioning for Mandibular Arch (Slides 14 through 19)

7. Producing Special Radiographs (Slide 20)

   a. Occlusal Radiographs

   b. Pediatric Radiographs

   c. Edentulous Radiographic Survey

   d. Endodontic Radiographic Technique

   e. Special Needs Patients/Compromised Patients

8. Processing Quality Radiographs (Slides 22 and 23)

9. Manual Processing Equipment

   a. Processing Preparation

   b. Manual Film Processing Technique

   c. Composition of Processing Solutions

10. Automatic Processing

11. Mounting Radiographs (Slide 24)

12. Radiographic Errors (Slides 25 through 36)

   a. Common Exposure Errors

      i. Distortion

      ii. Elongation

      iii. Foreshortening

      iv. Overlapping

     v. Cone cutting

     vi. Clear film/Absence of film

     vii. Double exposure

     viii. Blurred image

     ix. Underexposed film

     x. Overexposed film

     xi. Film artifacts

     xii. Backward film

  b. Common Film Processing Errors (Slides 38 through 42)

     i. Light film image

     ii. Dark film image

     iii. Fogged film

     iv. Partial image

     v. Spotted Films

     vi. Torn or scratched film

     vii. Air bubbles

     viii. Reticulation

     ix. Streaks

13. Duplicating Radiographs (Slide 44)

14. Storage of Patient Radiographs (Slide 45)

15. Legal Implications of Radiographs (Slide 46)

16. Quality Assurance (Slide 47)

TEACHING STRATEGIES

1. Chapter contents are presented in the PowerPoint slides, which are found in the Instructor Resources to Accompany Delmar's *Dental Assisting*.

2. The student must remember much of this chapter's content and then apply it in the clinical setting.

3. The students should read the chapter, and after the lecture should proceed to hands-on learning of various exposure techniques.

4. Show the Delmar Dental Assisting video on radiology.

5. Discuss the various techniques and then have the students practice on a mannequin.

6. Booklets and videos on how to produce dental x-rays can be purchase from Kodak. The booklet most pertinent to this chapter is *Producing Dental Radiographs*.

7. In the classroom, show various types of radiographs and discuss how they are exposed.

8. Using x-rays that the students have taken, discuss various errors. Give the students a picture of several different x-rays and have them label the errors.

CASE STUDY ANSWERS

1. Factors to consider include: reducing the exposure time and keeping the number of radiographs to a minimum because developing tissues are sensitive to radiation. The dental assistant needs to explain the procedure to the child and what they can expect, evaluate the child's ability to cooperate, and evaluate the child's mouth for sensitive areas.

2. For a 6-year old child the routine full mouth set of x-rays are twelve No. 0 size films including two bite-wings, six anterior incisors, and four posterior periapicals. The assistant determines if this needs to be altered by examining the child's mouth. The size of the patient's mouth will determine the size and number of films needed to view the information the dentist requested. One alternative is to take two occlusals films using No. 2 size films instead of the six No. 0 size anterior films.

3. Usually the anterior films are taken first to encourage the child's cooperation. These films are not as invasive and easier for the child to adapt to their placement.

4. At 6 years of age, Coral is still in the mixed dentition stage. She will probably have lost some primary teeth, have some permanent teeth at various stages of eruption, and have some loose teeth. The paralleling technique would be the most common and accurate technique to use on children.

TEXTBOOK REVIEW ANSWERS

Multiple Choice

1. a   2. b   3. d   4. c   5. b   6. a   7. a   8. b

9. c   10. b

Critical Thinking

1. The dental assistant would want to check the processing solutions to ensure that the chemicals are still effective and do not need changing. If the solutions are correct, then the films may be overexposed. The kV, mA, and electronic timer on the x-ray machine should be checked to verify that they are working properly. Also, check the package to determine whether the film is outdated, has been contaminated, and is being exposed and processed according to the manufacturer's directions.

2. Overlapping—adjust the horizontal angulation; cone cutting—adjust the position indicator device (PID) to cover the entire surface of the film; film placement—position the film correctly to expose the selected teeth in the radiograph and ensure that the patient maintains placement during exposure.

3. Films must be gently placed in the child's mouth because of developing tissues and loose or erupting teeth. The child's behavior and cooperation level must be evaluated and then an appropriate technique used to take the necessary radiographs. Various sizes of films may be required; in addition, the number may vary depending on what the dentist requires for diagnosis.

Extraoral and Digital Radiography

SPECIFIC INSTRUCTIONAL OBJECTIVES

1. Identify extraoral films and describe exposing techniques.

2. Identify normal and abnormal radiographic landmarks.

3. Identify imaging systems used for dental purposes.

4. Describe digital radiography.

5. Identify the components of digital radiography.

6. Explain the procedure for using digital radiography.

7. Describe 3-D imaging systems.

PREPARATORY

Personnel

Primary instructor who is knowledgeable about the dental profession and understands the information the dental assistant must know to become familiar with producing and evaluating dental radiographs. This instructor should be a Certified Dental Assistant with the radiology certificate if required by his or her state Dental Practice Act.

The number of students in a class will determine the number of instructors needed for this chapter because there are both lecture and clinical portions. In the clinical portion, the student requires hands-on instruction and learning activities that are better accomplished in smaller groups.

Suggested Audiovisual and Resource Materials

▶ *Workbook:* Chapter 23.

▶ *Delmar's Dental Assisting Video Series:* Appropriate content is available on Tape 2, *Dental Radiography.* This includes exposing radiographs.

▶ *Image Library:* Provides illustrations from Chapter 23 of the textbook that can be used via computer or as transparencies to provide visual support for classroom instruction.

▶ *Computerized Test Bank:* Provides additional test questions for Chapter 23 and related material on the DANB examination.

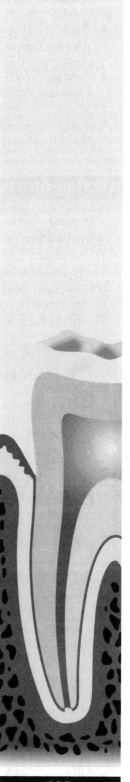

▶ **Practice Software:** Additional practice exercises that further reinforce Chapter 23 content can be found on the software disk that accompanies this textbook.

▶ **Interactive Skills CD:** Radiographs.

▶ **Dental Terminology, Third Edition:** Chapter 9, Radiography.

▶ **Dental Assisting Coloring Book:** Chapters 9 and 10—Dental X-Ray and Film Holding Devices, and Radiology Landmarks.

▶ **Delmar's Dental Assisting Exam Review:** Additional review material, test questions, and rationale provide practice for the DANB examination.

▶ **CourseMate:** Additional practice exercises that further reinforce Chapter 23 content can be found on the CourseMate Web site.

▶ **Recommended minimum time to complete Chapter 23:** 5 to 6 hours, depending on depth of information the instructor wishes to cover and the skill level required by students.

LECTURE OUTLINE CORRELATED TO INSTRUCTOR PRESENTATIONS IN POWERPOINT

The presentations provided contain lecture notes. The notes can be viewed in PowerPoint when viewing the slides in either the normal or outline view. To print the slides with the notes: From your print box look for the "Print What" and change the drop-down to "Notes Pages." A new feature called "Dental Checks" has been interspersed throughout the presentations to keep the student engaged in the materials during the lecture. This feature contains a quick question followed by the answer to stimulate a brief discussion.

1. Extraoral Radiographs (Slide 2)

   a. Panoramic Radiography (Slides 3 through 6)

      i. Fundamentals of Panoramic Radiography

      ii. Panoramic Unit

      iii. Panoramic Exposure Technique Suggestions

      iv. Common Panoramic Radiography Errors

   b. Cephalometric Radiographs (Slide 8)

2. Radiographic Interpretation (Slide 9)

   a. Tooth and Surrounding Tissues (Slide 10)

   b. Mandibular Landmarks (Slide 11)

   c. Maxillary Landmarks (Slide 12)

3. Imaging Systems/Digital Imaging Systems (Slide 13)

   a. Computed Tomography (CT Scanning)

   b. Magnetic Resonance Imaging

4. Digital Radiography in the Dental Office (Slides 14 through 18)

   a. Fundamental Concepts of Digital Radiography

   b. Types of Digital Imaging

    c. Digital Radiography Equipment

    d. Advantages and Disadvantages of Digital Radiography

5. 3-Dimensional Imaging in Dentistry (Slides 19 through 21)

    a. CBVT and CBVI

    b. Use of 3-D Imaging

       i. Endodontics

       ii. Periodontics

       iii. Orthodontics

       iv. Maxillofacial surgery

       v. General dentistry

    c. Benefits of 3-D Imaging

    d. Patient Preparation

6. Hand-Held Intraoral Radiography (Slide 22)

TEACHING STRATEGIES

1. Chapter contents are presented in the PowerPoint slides, which are found in the Instructor Resources to Accompany Delmar's *Dental Assisting*.

2. Much of the content in this chapter must be remembered by the student and then applied in the clinical setting.

3. Students should read the chapter, and after the lecture proceed to hands-on practice to learn the various extraoral radiographs and digital radiography.

4. Booklets and video on how to expose panoramic radiographs can be purchased from Kodak. The most pertinent for this chapter is *Panoramic Radiographs*.

5. In the classroom, demonstrate panoramic film and a cassette and discuss how this film is exposed.

6. If you have a panoramic machine in your dental clinic, demonstrate to the students the technique for exposing a panoramic radiograph. If you do not have a panoramic machine, arrange to visit a dental office or clinic to demonstrate taking panoramic exposures.

7. After the students have exposed a panoramic radiograph, have them bring it to class. Review landmarks with them and have the students mark the landmarks on the panoramic x-ray.

8. Digital radiography also requires similar hands-on demonstrations. Student learning depends on available equipment. Dental equipment sales representatives may be helpful in this regard.

9. Training videos are available for all digital radiography systems. Show one of these in the classroom and then review the steps of exposure with the students.

10. Have the students complete the "Matching" exercise.

CASE STUDY ANSWERS

1. Digital radiology technology is becoming popular in many dental offices. The technology is advancing as more and more dental professionals decide to switch to digital.

2. Advantages include less exposure to radiation for patients, immediate results, and the ability to enhance the digital exposure, provide visual images for the patient, store images for future or immediate reference, and send digital images to other dental offices and insurance companies. In addition, digital technology does not require processing equipment and supplies. Disadvantages include initial expense of the equipment and software, time required to learn the system and become proficient, sensors that are sometimes uncomfortable for patient placement and exposure, technology compatibility concerns about storage and transferring to updated systems, the possibility of computer viruses, and so forth.

3. When a dentist decides to switch to digital imaging radiography, there is a learning curve for the technology. Staff members need to learn the software as well as sensor usage. The dentist must be willing to allow time for training and practice to achieve the expected quality that digital radiography can provide.

TEXTBOOK REVIEW ANSWERS

Multiple Choice

1. d   2. a   3. c   4. b   5. c   6. b   7. c   8. d

9. b   10. b

Critical Thinking

1. The panoramic x-ray would be the most likely to be requested. An occlusal radiograph could also be used if the patient could be positioned correctly. The dental assistant would be able to obtain the panoramic radiograph.

2. A panoramic radiograph will show all the landmarks listed.

3. Both intraoral films and extraoral films can be taken with digital imaging. This includes periapical, bite wings, occlusals, panoramic, cephalometric, and 3D imaging. The advantages of digital imaging include:

   ▶ Less exposure to radiation for the patient.

   ▶ Images appear almost immediately after exposure.

   ▶ The images can be enhanced for better interpretation and evaluation.

   ▶ Patients can view the images as the dentist explains areas of concern.

   ▶ Images are stored on the computer.

   ▶ Eliminates need for darkroom and processing equipment.

   ▶ Digital images can be sent electronically to other dental offices, insurance companies, patients, etc.

   ▶ Techniques are becoming easier to learn and sensors/imaging plates are becoming more comfortable for patients.

Endodontics

SPECIFIC INSTRUCTIONAL OBJECTIVES

1. Define endodontics and describe what an endodontist does.

2. Describe pulpal and periapical disease.

3. Identify diagnostic procedures.

4. Identify instruments used in endodontic procedures and describe their functions.

5. Identify materials used in endodontics and describe their functions.

6. Describe endodontic procedures and the responsibilities of the dental assistant.

7. Describe endodontic retreatment.

8. Explain surgical endodontic procedures and the instruments used.

PREPARATORY

Personnel

Primary instructor who is knowledgeable about the dental profession and understands the information the dental assistant requires about endodontics as a specialty and endodontic procedures completed in the general dental office. This instructor should be a Certified Dental Assistant.

The number of students in a class will determine the number of instructors needed for this chapter because there are both lecture and clinical portions. In the clinical portion, the student requires hands-on instruction and learning activities that are better accomplished in smaller groups.

Suggested Audiovisual and Resource Materials

▶ *Workbook:* Chapter 24.

▶ *Image Library:* Provides illustrations from Chapter 24 of the textbook that can be used via computer or as transparencies to provide visual support for classroom instruction.

▶ *Computerized Test Bank:* Provides additional test questions for Chapter 24 and related material on the DANB examination.

▶ *Practice Software:* Additional practice exercises that further reinforce Chapter 24 content can be found on the software disk that accompanies this textbook.

▶ *Interactive Skills CD:* Specialty Setups: Endodontics.

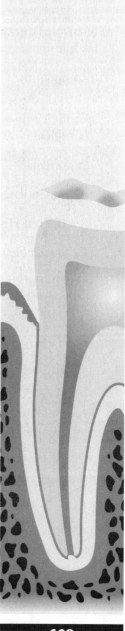

◗ *Dental Terminology, Third Edition:* Chapter 13, Endodontics.

◗ *Delmar's Dental Assisting Exam Review:* Additional review material, test questions, and rationales provide practice for the DANB examination.

◗ *Dental Assisting Instrument Guide:* Review of instrumentation used in endodontic procedures.

◗ *CourseMate:* Additional practice exercises that further reinforce Chapter 24 content can be found on the CourseMate Web site.

◗ *Recommended minimum time to complete Chapter 24:* 6 to 8 hours, depending on depth of information the instructor wishes to cover and the skill level required by students.

LECTURE OUTLINE CORRELATED TO INSTRUCTOR PRESENTATIONS IN POWERPOINT

The presentations provided contain lecture notes. The notes can be viewed in PowerPoint when viewing the slides in either the normal or outline view. To print the slides with the notes: From your print box look for the "Print What" and change the drop-down to "Notes Pages," A new feature called "Dental Checks" has been interspersed throughout the presentations to keep the student engaged in the materials during the lecture. This feature contains a quick question followed by the answer to stimulate a brief discussion.

1. Endodontic Team (Slide 2)

2. Progress of Pulpal and Periapical Diseases (Slides 3 and 4)

    a. Pulpal Diseases (Slides 5 through 10)

    b. Periapical Diseases (Slides 11 through 13)

3. Endodontic Diagnosis (Slide 14)

    a. Medical History (Slide 15)

    b. Dental History (Slide 16)

    c. Clinical Examination and Pulp Testing (Slides 17 through 22)

        i. Radiographs

        ii. Palpation

        iii. Percussion

        iv. Mobility

        v. Cold test

        vi. Heat test

        vii. Electric pulp testing/vitality scanner

        viii. Transillumination test

        ix. Selective anesthesia

        x. Caries removal

    d. Treatment Plan

4. Endodontic Instruments (Slides 24 through 37)

    a. Characteristics of Intracanal Instruments

    b. Barbed Broaches

    c. Files

    d. Reamers

    e. Rotary Intracanal Instruments

    f. Endodontic Organizers

    g. Rubber Stops

    h. Gates-Glidden Drills

    i. Peeso Reamers

    j. Lentulo Spirals

    k. Endodontic Spoon Excavator

    l. Endodontic Explorer

    m. Endodontic Spreaders, Pluggers, and the Glick #1

5. Endodontic Materials (Slides 39 through 42)

    a. Absorbent Paper Points

    b. Gutta Percha

    c. Irrigation Solutions

    d. Root Canal Disinfecting, Cleaning, and Lubricating

    e. Root Canal Sealers/Cements

6. Equipment Used in Endodontic Procedures (Slide 43)

    a. Apex finder

    b. Heating unit

    c. Endodontic handpiece

    d. Ultrasonic unit

    e. Endodontic bender

    f. Dental microscope

    g. Endodontic obturation system

7. Sterilization Procedures

8. Endodontic Procedures

    a. Root Canal Treatment (Slides 44 through 46)

    b. Endodontic Retreatment (Slides 47 and 48)

    c. Pulpectomy (Slide 49)

    d. Pulpotomy (Slides 50 and 51)

9. Surgical Endodontics (Slide 52)

    a. Apicoectomy (Slide 53)

    b. Root Amputation (Slide 54)

    c. Hemisection (Slide 55)

    d. Apexification (Slide 56)

    e. Apexogenesis (Slide 57)

TEACHING STRATEGIES

1. Chapter contents are presented in the PowerPoint slides, which are found in the Instructor Resources to Accompany Delmar's *Dental Assisting*.

2. Much of the content in this chapter must be remembered by the student and then applied in the clinical setting.

3. The students should read the chapter, complete the assignment in Chapter 24 of the Workbook, and then proceed to hands-on practice to learn the endodontic instruments and procedures.

4. Have the students use Delmar's *Dental Assisting Instrument Guide* to assist in learning endodontic instruments and equipment.

5. Invite an endodontist as a guest speaker to the class.

CASE STUDY ANSWERS

1. The key indications for treatment are that Mr. Frank is experiencing pain and there is inflammation.

2. The clinical tests the dental assistant should prepare may include an x-ray of the area, an electric pulp test, thermal pulp testing, mobility testing, and possible selective anesthesia.

3. The probable treatment is a root canal if the clinical test indicates inflamed or nonvital pulp.

4. Mr. Frank should be informed about the condition of the tooth and possible treatment options.

TEXTBOOK REVIEW ANSWERS

Multiple Choice

1. d	2. d	3. b	4. c	5. b	6. b	7. a	8. a
9. a	10. c						

Critical Thinking

1. A pulpectomy involves removing the pulp chamber and part of the root canal. A pulpotomy involves removing the pulp in the pulp chamber. A root canal treatment involves complete removal of the pulp from a tooth.

2. No, anesthetic is not always administered for root canal treatment. If there is pulpal necrosis and the tooth has been opened and allowed to drain, the patient should experience no pain during treatment.

3. K-type files are tightly twisted; Hedström files are manufactured through a different process and are shaped like a stack of cones.

Oral and Maxillofacial Surgery

SPECIFIC INSTRUCTIONAL OBJECTIVES

1. Describe the scope of oral and maxillofacial surgery.

2. Identify the surgical instruments used in various types of surgery and describe their functions.

3. Explain the aseptic procedures followed in the oral surgeon's office.

4. Describe evaluation procedures for new patients.

5. Describe how to prepare the patient for surgical treatment.

6. Explain surgical procedures, including tray setups and assisting responsibilities.

7. List the postoperative instructions given to patients.

8. List and describe cancer and oral abnormalities detection.

9. List and describe biopsy techniques.

10. Describe temporomandibular joint (TMJ) disease.

11. List and describe the types of dental implants and explain the surgical procedures for placing the implants.

12. Explain the oral surgeon's relationship with the hospital.

Advanced Chairside Functions

13. Explain the function of sutures and when they are placed.

14. List the equipment and supplies needed for suture removal.

15. Determine and identify the location and number of sutures and how to evaluate the healing process.

16. Identify the following suture patterns: simple, continuous simple, sling, continuous sling, horizontal, and vertical mattress.

17. List the basic criteria for suture removal.

18. Explain the steps of removal for identified suture patterns.

19. Explain postoperative patient care.

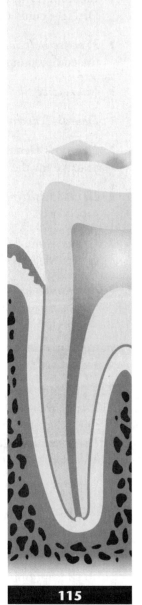

Personnel

Primary instructor who is knowledgeable of the dental profession and understands the information the dental assistant needs to know about oral maxillofacial surgery as a specialty and selected procedures that are completed in the general dental office. This instructor should be a Certified Dental Assistant.

The number of students in a class will determine the number of instructors required for this topic because there are both lecture and clinical portions. In the clinical portion, the student requires hands-on instruction and learning activities that are better accomplished in small groups.

Suggested Audiovisual and Resource Materials

▶ *Workbook:* Chapter 25.

▶ *Image Library:* Provides illustrations from Chapter 25 of the textbook that can be used via computer or as transparencies to provide visual support for classroom instruction.

▶ *Computerized Test Bank:* Provides additional test questions for Chapter 25 and related material on the DANB examination.

▶ *Practice Software:* Additional practice exercises that further reinforce Chapter 25 content can be found on the companion software disk.

▶ *Interactive Skills CD:* Specialty Setups: Oral Surgery.

▶ *Dental Terminology, Third Edition:* Chapter 14, Oral and Maxillofacial Surgery.

▶ *Delmar's Dental Assisting Exam Review:* Additional review material, test questions, and rationales provide practice for the DANB examination.

▶ *Dental Assisting Instrument Guide:* Review of instrumentation used in oral and maxillofacial surgery procedures.

▶ *CourseMate:* Additional practice exercises that further reinforce Chapter 25 content can be found on the CourseMate Web site.

▶ *Recommended minimum time to complete Chapter 25:* 6 to 8 hours, depending on depth of information the instructor wishes to cover and the skill level required by students.

LECTURE OUTLINE CORRELATED TO INSTRUCTOR PRESENTATIONS IN POWERPOINT

The presentations provided contain lecture notes. The notes can be viewed in PowerPoint when viewing the slides in either the normal or outline view. To print the slides with the notes: From your print box look for the "Print What" and change the drop-down to "Notes Pages." A new feature called "Dental Checks" has been interspersed throughout the presentations to keep the student engaged in the materials during the lecture. This feature contains a quick question followed by the answer to stimulate a brief discussion.

1. The Oral and Maxillofacial Surgeon's Office (Slide 2)

2. The Oral and Maxillofacial Surgery Team (Slide 3)

    a. Oral and Maxillofacial Surgeon

    b. Receptionist and Business Staff

    c. Surgical Dental Assistant

    d. Nurse Anesthetist or Anesthesiologist

3. Oral Surgery Instruments (Slides 4 through 21)

    a. Scalpel

    b. Retractors

    c. Mouth Props

    d. Hemostats

    e. Needle Holders

    f. Surgical Scissors

    g. Surgical Aspirating Tips

    h. Surgical Curettes

    i. Surgical Chisels and Mallets

    j. Rongeurs

    k. Surgical Bone Files

    l. Periosteal Elevator

    m. Elevators

    n. Forceps

4. Asepsis in Oral Surgery (Slide 23)

5. Patient Considerations (Slide 24)

6. Patient Preparation

7. Oral Surgery Procedures

    a. Routine or Uncomplicated Extractions (Slides 25 and 26)

    b. Multiple Extractions and Alveoplasty (Slides 27 and 28)

    c. Impacted Teeth Extractions (Slides 29 through 33)

    d. Cancer and Oral Abnormalities Detection (Slide 34)

    e. Biopsy Procedures (Slides 35 through 39)

    f. Dental Implant Surgery (Slides 40 through 43)

8. Postoperative Care of the Patient (Slide 44)

9. Postsurgical Complications (Slides 45 through 47)

10. Temporomandibular Joint Disease (Slides 48 through 53)

    a. Signs and Symptoms of TMJ Dysfunction

    b. Diagnosing TMJ Dysfunction

    c. Treatment Options for TMJ Dysfunction

11. Hospital Dentistry (Slide 54)

12. Advanced Chairside Functions (Slides 55 and 56)

    a. Suture Removal

        i. Procedures Prior to Removal of Sutures

        ii. Prepare Suture Removal Equipment and Supplies

        iii. Review the Patient's Chart

        iv. Examine the Suture Site

        v. Consult with the Dentist

    b. Types of Suture Patterns

        i. Simple Suture

        ii. Continuous Simple Suture

        iii. Sling Suture

        iv. Continuous Sling Suture

        v. Mattress Sutures

    c. Suture Removal Criteria

    d. Post-Suture Removal

TEACHING STRATEGIES

1. Chapter contents are presented in the PowerPoint slides, which are found in the Instructor Resources to Accompany Delmar's *Dental Assisting.*

2. Much of the content in this chapter must be remembered by the student for application in the clinical setting.

3. Students should read the chapter and complete the assignment in the workbook, followed by hands-on practice to learn the oral surgery instruments and various procedures.

4. Have the students use *Delmar's Dental Assisting Instrument Guide* to assist in their learning the oral surgery instruments.

5. Demonstrate to the class how to do a surgical scrub and have the students practice the technique.

6. Removing sutures is included in this section, and the students need to practice this skill. Ask the dentist to tie several different types of sutures and then, after giving detailed instructions, have the students remove them and explain the technique.

7. Have the students role-play giving home-care instructions to a patient who has just had all four impacted wisdom teeth removed.

8. Invite an oral maxillofacial surgeon as a guest speaker to the class.

CASE STUDY ANSWERS

1. Mr. Scott would make an appointment with an oral surgeon to evaluate whether there is adequate alveolar bone.

2. Dental implants provide an option to a dental bridge or partial denture.

3. The dental assistant would need to prepare the operatory, sterilize the necessary instruments, and prepare the examination tray.

4. An oral maxillofacial surgeon, a general dentist, and/or a prosthodontist would be involved in Mr. Scott's treatment.

TEXTBOOK REVIEW ANSWERS

Multiple Choice

1. b   2. c   3. a   4. c   5. d   6. b   7. c   8. a

9. c   10. c

Critical Thinking

1. The maxillary forceps must adapt to the root anatomy of the maxillary molars, which have three roots—two on the buccal and one on the lingual. The mandibular forceps can be used on the left or right quadrants because the mandibular molars have two roots.

2. The patient does not have to be without teeth at all. Before the last teeth are extracted, impressions are taken and an immediate denture is made. Once the teeth are extracted and the bone and tissue contoured, the immediate denture is put in the patient's mouth, so the patient is never without teeth. Other options would involve a time when the patient would be without teeth. Sometimes a patient will have their teeth extracted and then wait until the bone and tissues heal before having a denture made.

3. The basic responsibilities of the surgical assistant are evacuating with a surgical high volume evacuation tip, maintaining a clear view for the oral surgeon, retraction of tissues, transferring instruments, caring for the patient before and after surgery, and maintaining a sterile field. These responsibilities may change if there is a second assistant and the duties are divided. The assistant must always be prepared for an emergency, where they would step up to assist the dentist in providing immediate care for the patient. With some procedures the assistant may be asked to prepare materials and/or specific items needed, such as dental implants, burs, etc.

4. There are many variations as to when the dentist actually is called to examine the patient. The dentist may examine the patient before the assistant removes the sutures, or after the sutures have been removed. How the tissues have healed at the wound site determines what is going to be done and when the dentist examines the site. The dental assistant must keep the dentist informed of the patient's status when removing sutures.

5. The dental assistant may ask the patient the following questions and then relay the information to the dentist:

   Do you experience popping and clicking noises when opening your mouth?

   Is the pain you are experiencing located around your ears?

   Do you clench your teeth or tighten your jaw muscles?

6. Dental implants are a good treatment choice if the patient has little bone to support a denture or a partial. Dental implants replace one tooth or several teeth without disturbing adjacent teeth.

CHAPTER **26**

Oral Pathology

SPECIFIC INSTRUCTIONAL OBJECTIVES

1. Define oral pathology and identify the dental assistant's role in this specialty.

2. Characterize the process of inflammation.

3. Identify oral lesions according to placement.

4. Identify oral diseases and lesions related to biological agents.

5. Describe oral diseases and lesions related to physical agents.

6. Identify oral diseases and lesions related to chemical agents.

7. Identify oral conditions related to hormonal disturbances.

8. Identify oral conditions related to developmental disturbances.

9. Distinguish among oral conditions related to nutritional deficiencies.

10. Identify the conditions and lesions of oral neoplasms.

11. Identify oral lesions related to HIV and AIDS.

12. Describe the conditions related to miscellaneous disorders affecting the oral cavity.

PREPARATORY

Personnel

Instructors who teach dental pathology should have a dental assisting or science background, with knowledge of pathogens that affect the oral cavity.

Suggested Audiovisual and Resource Materials

▶ *Workbook:* Chapter 26.

▶ *Image Library:* Provides illustrations from Chapter 26 of the textbook that can be used via computer or as transparencies to provide visual support for classroom instruction.

▶ *Computerized Test Bank:* Provides additional test questions for Chapter 26 and related material on the DANB examination.

▶ *Practice Software:* Additional practice exercises that further reinforce Chapter 26 content can be found on the companion software disk.

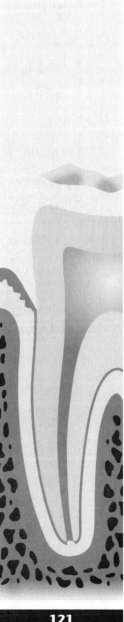

▶ *Delmar's Dental Assisting Exam Review:* Additional review material, test questions, and rationales provide practice for the DANB examination.

▶ *CourseMate:* Additional practice exercises that further reinforce Chapter 26 content can be found on the CourseMate Web site.

▶ *Recommended minimum time to complete Chapter 26:* 5 to 6 hours, depending on depth of information the instructor wishes to cover.

LECTURE OUTLINE CORRELATED TO INSTRUCTOR PRESENTATIONS IN POWERPOINT

The presentations provided contain lecture notes. The notes can be viewed in PowerPoint when viewing the slides in either the normal or outline view. To print the slides with the notes: From your print box look for the "Print What" and change the drop-down to "Notes Pages." A new feature called "Dental Checks" has been interspersed throughout the presentations to keep the student engaged in the materials during the lecture. This feature contains a quick question followed by the answer to stimulate a brief discussion.

1. Inflammation (Slide 4)

    a. Redness

    b. Heat

    c. Swelling

    d. Pain

2. Diagnosing Oral Pathology (Slide 5)

3. Oral Lesions (Slides 6 through 10)

    a. Above-Surface Lesions

        i. Blister

        ii. Bulla

        iii. Hematoma

        iv. Papule

        v. Plaque

        vi. Pustule

        vii. Vesicle

    b. Below-Surface Lesions

        i. Abscess

        ii. Cyst

        iii. Erosion

        iv. Ulcer

    c. Even or Flat with Surface Lesions

        i. Ecchymosis

        ii. Macule

        iii. Patch

        iv. Petechiae

        v. Purpura

    d. Flat or Above-Surface Lesions

        i. Granuloma

        ii. Neoplasm

        iii. Nodule

4. Biological Agents (Slides 12 through 14)

    a. Actinomycosis

    b. Herpes Simplex

    c. Aphthous Ulcers

    d. Herpes Zoster

    e. Syphilis

    f. Thrush

5. Physical Agents (Slides 15 through 17)

    a. Denture Irritation Causing Hyperplasia

    b. Amalgam Tattoo

    c. Radiation Injury

    d. Oral Piercing

    e. Tongue Splitting

6. Chemical Agents (Slides 19 through 21)

    a. Aspirin Burn

    b. Nicotine Stomatitis

    c. Chewing Tobacco (Snuff) Lesion

    d. Hairy Tongue

    e. Gingival Hyperplasia

    f. Meth Mouth

7. Hormonal Disturbances (Slide 22)

   a. Pregnancy Gingivitis

   b. Pyogenic Granuloma

   c. Puberty Gingival Enlargement

8. Developmental Disturbances (Slides 23 through 31)

   a. Disturbances in Tooth Development

      i. Amelogenesis imperfecta

      ii. Ankylosis

      iii. Anodontia

      iv. Dentinogenesis imperfecta

      v. Fusion

      vi. Gemination

      vii. Macrodontia

      viii. Microdontia

      ix. Neonatal teeth

      x. Supernumerary teeth

      xi. Twinning

   b. Oral Tori

   c. Exostoses

   d. Fordyce's Spots (Granules)

   e. Fissured Tongue

   f. Bifid Tongue

   g. Ankyloglossia

9. Nutritional Disturbances (Slide 33)

   a. Angular Cheilitis

   b. Glossitis (Bald Tongue)

10. Neoplasms (Slides 34 through 41)

   a. Leukoplakia

   b. Lichen Planus

   c. Erythroplakia

   d. Squamous Cell Carcinoma

    e. Basal Cell Carcinoma

    f. Papilloma

    g. Fibroma

11. Oral Lesions Related to HIV and AIDS (Slides 42 and 43)

    a. Hairy Leukoplakia

    b. *Candida albicans*

    c. Kaposi's Sarcoma

12. Miscellaneous Disorders (Slides 44 through 46)

    a. Acute Necrotizing Ulcerative Gingivitis

    b. Mucocele

    c. Varix

    d. Geographic Tongue

    e. Anorexia Nervosa and Bulimia

    f. Bell's Palsy

TEACHING STRATEGIES

1. Chapter contents are presented in the PowerPoint slides, which are found in the Instructor Resources to Accompany Delmar's *Dental Assisting*.

2. Pictures are useful when learning about oral lesions. Many pictures are provided in the textbook and PowerPoint slides. Others can be obtained online or direct from dental schools, dentists, and the American Dental Association. When talking about each lesion, show a picture and give the information.

3. Much of the information in this chapter should be memorized. Consider providing students with a memory-reinforcement study guide that requires them to write out terminology.

4. In a quiz, reproduce photos in the workbook and have students label them.

5. Showing students case studies and talking about them will give the students an understanding of how the dentist approaches the diagnosis. It will also show them that several diagnoses are possible, and that only through biopsy and other tests can the diagnosis be confirmed.

CASE STUDY ANSWERS

1. The pathologic condition in Toby's mouth is a hematoma.

2. The dental assistant should alert the dentist, and then apply pressure to the area.

3. The prognosis of this condition is that when pressure is applied to this area, the blood will disperse into the tissue, which will alleviate the pressure in the area.

TEXTBOOK REVIEW ANSWERS

Multiple Choice

1. b	2. d	3. d	4. b	5. d	6. d	7. b	8. d

9. c   10. b

Critical Thinking

1. A torus mandibularis is not a serious condition. It is seen in approximately one in every five adults. While taking the radiographs, the dental assistant should take care not to abrade the tissue covering the bony growth.

2. Vitamin B–complex deficiency may cause glossitis (bald tongue). The tongue may be sore, but diet modification will help correct this condition.

3. The warning signs of oral cancer are a sore in the oral cavity that does not heal in a month; lumps and swelling in the oral cavity or on the lips or neck; white or rough lesions in the mouth or on the lips; mouth dryness over time for no apparent reason; numbness in or around the oral cavity; soreness or burning sensation in or around the oral cavity; and difficulty speaking, eating, or swallowing.

Orthodontics

SPECIFIC INSTRUCTIONAL OBJECTIVES

1. Define orthodontics and describe the orthodontic setting.

2. Define the role of the dental assistant in an orthodontic setting.

3. Define and describe occlusion and malocclusion.

4. Identify the causes of malocclusion.

5. Describe preventive, interceptive, and corrective orthodontics.

6. Explain the process of tooth movement.

7. Describe the preorthodontic appointment for diagnostic records.

8. Describe the consultation appointment and the roles of the assistant, patient, and orthodontist.

9. Differentiate between fixed and removable appliances.

10. Identify and describe the function of basic orthodontic instruments.

11. Describe the stages of orthodontic treatment.

12. Explain the procedure for removing orthodontic appliances and how the teeth are retained in position after appliance removal.

PREPARATORY

Personnel

Primary instructor who is knowledgeable of the dental profession and understands the information the dental assistant needs to know about orthodontics as a specialty. This instructor should be a Certified Dental Assistant and if possible a Certified Orthodontic Assistant.

The number of students in a class will determine the number of instructors required for this topic because there are both lecture and clinical portions. In the clinical portion, the student requires hands-on instruction and learning activities that are better accomplished in small groups.

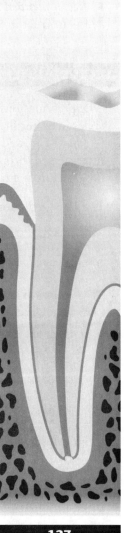

Suggested Audiovisual and Resource Materials

▶ *Workbook:* Chapter 27.

▶ *Image Library:* Provides illustrations from Chapter 27 of the textbook that can be used via computer or as transparencies to provide visual support for classroom instruction.

▶ *Computerized Test Bank:* Provides additional test questions for Chapter 27 and related material on the DANB examination.

▶ *Practice Software:* Additional practice exercises that further reinforce Chapter 27 content can be found on the companion software disk.

▶ *Interactive Skills CD:* Specialty Setups: Orthodontics.

▶ *Dental Terminology, Third Edition:* Chapter 15, Orthodontics.

▶ *Delmar's Dental Assisting Exam Review:* Additional review material, test questions, and rationales provide practice for the DANB examination.

▶ *Dental Assisting Instrument Guide:* Review of instrumentation used in orthodontics.

▶ *CourseMate:* Additional practice exercises that further reinforce Chapter 27 content can be found on the CourseMate Web site.

▶ *Recommended minimum time to complete Chapter 27:* 5 to 8 hours, depending on depth of information the instructor wishes to cover and the skill level required by students.

LECTURE OUTLINE CORRELATED TO INSTRUCTOR PRESENTATIONS IN POWERPOINT

The presentations provided contain lecture notes. The notes can be viewed in PowerPoint when viewing the slides in either the normal or outline view. To print the slides with the notes: From your print box look for the "Print What" and change the drop-down to "Notes Pages." A new feature called "Dental Checks" has been interspersed throughout the presentations to keep the student engaged in the materials during the lecture. This feature contains a quick question followed by the answer to stimulate a brief discussion.

1. The Orthodontic Practice (Slide 3)

    a. Office

    b. Team

2. Occlusion and Malocclusion (Slides 5 through 10)

    a. Normal Occlusion

    b. Malocclusion

3. Malpositions of Individual Teeth and Groups of Teeth (Slides 11 through 16)

    a. Torsoversion

    b. Mesioversion

    c. Distoversion

      d. Linguoversion

      e. Labioversion

      f. Supraversion

      g. Infraversion

      h. Transversion

4. Etiology of Malocclusion (Slide 17)

      a. Genetic or hereditary

      b. Systemic

      c. Local

5. Types of Orthodontic Treatments (Slide 19)

      a. Preventive and Interceptive Orthodontics

      b. Corrective Orthodontics

6. Process of Tooth Movement (Slides 20 and 21)

7. Preorthodontic Treatment (Slide 22)

      a. Diagnostic Records

      b. Medical–Dental History

      c. Clinical Examination

      d. Radiographs (Slide 23)

      e. Photographs

      f. Study Models

8. Consultation Appointment (Slide 24)

9. Orthodontic Appliances (Slides 25 through 30)

      a. Fixed Appliances

         i. Bands

        ii. Brackets

       iii. Arch wires

       iv. Ligature wire, rings, ties, chains

        v. Buccal tubes

       vi. Springs

      vii. Elastics

    b. Special Fixed Appliances

        i. Lingual braces

        ii. Lingual arch wire

        iii. Space maintainer

        iv. Palatal expanding appliance

    c. Removable Appliances

        i. Headgear

        ii. Functional appliances

        iii. Retainers

        iv. Tooth positioner

        v. Esthetic orthodontic aligners

10. Three-Dimensional Imaging in Orthodontics (Slide 32)

11. Orthodontic Instruments (Slides 33 through 41)

12. Orthodontic Treatment (Slides 42 through 45)

    a. Separators

    b. Selection of Orthodontic Bands

    c. Band Cementation

    d. Direct Bonding Brackets

    e. Placement of Arch Wire

    f. Oral Hygiene Instructions

    g. Periodic Office Visits for Adjustments

13. Completion Appointment (Slides 46 through 48)

TEACHING STRATEGIES

1. Chapter contents are presented in the PowerPoint slides, which are found in the Instructor Resources to Accompany Delmar's *Dental Assisting*.

2. Much of the content in this chapter must be remembered by the student for application in the clinical setting.

   Students should read the chapter and complete the assignment in the workbook followed by hands-on practice to learn the orthodontic instruments and various procedures.

3. Have the students use *Delmar's Dental Assisting Instrument Guide* to assist in learning the orthodontic instruments.

4. Have students who have had orthodontic treatment share their experience with the class.

5. Provide models of various malocclusion classifications, and have the students identify the classification of each. Using study models of their own teeth, ask students to identify their own occlusion and any maloccluded teeth.

6. Invite an orthodontist as a guest speaker to the class.

CASE STUDY ANSWERS

1. The dental assistant should prepare to take the patient's medical and dental history, panoramic and cephalometric x-rays, intraoral and facial photographs, and impressions for study models, and should prepare an examination tray set.

2. Yes, Chaz's age is a factor because his jaws are still developing.

3. Chaz is 12 years old and normally would have lost most of his primary teeth. His anterior teeth should be present or erupting. The cuspids may be erupting. His premolars and first molars should be present and the second molars should be erupting.

4. Chaz is a Class II Division 1 of Dr. Angle's classes of malocclusion.

TEXTBOOK REVIEW ANSWERS

Multiple Choice

1. d	2. c	3. c	4. a	5. c	6. b	7. a	8. d
9. c	10. c						

Critical Thinking

1. Answers will vary depending on the individual. Teeth might be linguoversion, mesioversion, distoversion, torsoversion, labioversion, supraversion, or infraversion.

2. Sticky foods, crunchy foods, and gum. Some crunchy foods, such as carrots and apples, can be eaten if cut into small pieces.

3. Genetic, systemic, and local. Genetic—supernumerary teeth, facial and palatal clefts, abnormal jaw relationships, or congenitally missing teeth. Systemic—diseases or nutritional disturbances of developing dentition. Local—trauma, thumb-sucking, tongue-sucking, mouth breathing, bruxism, or nail-biting.

4. Sometimes primary teeth are lost prematurely. It is important to maintain this space until the permanent tooth begins to erupt. If the space is not held open, the adjacent teeth will drift in and begin to fill the space, making it more difficult for the permanent tooth to come in straight.

    The space maintainer must be cemented in place to hold the teeth in position, and if it comes out it should be replaced as soon as possible to prevent the teeth from moving. If it is left out too long a new space maintainer must be fabricated.

5. Helping patients remain motivated to keep up their oral hygiene can sometimes be a challenge. Dental assistants are often in charge of this task. Educating the patient is the first step, followed by various techniques for brushing and flossing with braces in place. Each orthodontist has different ways to motivate and reward the patients who maintain good oral hygiene, including verbal and written encouragement; prizes, gift cards, passes to movies, and so on; and including patients in drawings for a more valuable prize.

Pediatric Dentistry and Enamel Sealants

SPECIFIC INSTRUCTIONAL OBJECTIVES

1. Define pediatric dentistry as a specialty.

2. Describe the pediatric office and team members.

3. Explain the common behavior characteristics of children of various ages.

4. Describe child behavior management techniques.

5. Explain the role of the parent or guardian in pediatric dentistry.

6. Identify common procedures in pediatric dentistry.

7. Identify the equipment unique to pediatric dentistry.

8. Explain common emergencies in pediatric dentistry and the treatment for these emergencies.

9. Identify the signs of child abuse and the procedure for reporting suspected child abuse cases.

Advanced Chairside Functions

10. Explain the purpose of using dental sealants and where they are placed.

11. List the indications and contraindications of placing sealants.

12. Discuss the role of the dental assistant in the placement of dental sealants.

13. Describe the types of sealant materials.

14. List and describe the steps of the application procedure.

PREPARATORY

Personnel

Primary instructor who is knowledgeable of the dental profession and understands the information the dental assistant needs to know about pediatric dentistry as a specialty and placing enamel sealants. This instructor should be a Certified Dental Assistant.

The number of students in a class will determine the number of instructors required for this topic because there are both lecture and clinical portions. In the clinical portion, the student requires hands-on instruction and learning activities that are better accomplished in small groups.

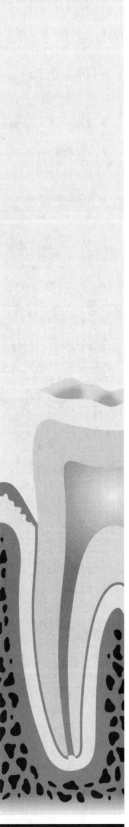

Suggested Audiovisual and Resource Materials

▶ *Workbook:* Chapter 28.

▶ *Image Library:* Provides illustrations from Chapter 28 of the textbook that can be used via computer or as transparencies to provide visual support for classroom instruction.

▶ *Computerized Test Bank:* Provides additional test questions for Chapter 28 and related material on the DANB examination.

▶ *Practice Software:* Additional practice exercises that further reinforce Chapter 28 content can be found on the companion software disk.

▶ *Dental Terminology, Third Edition:* Chapter 17, Pediatric Dentistry.

▶ *Delmar's Dental Assisting Exam Review:* Additional review material, test questions, and rationales provide practice for the DANB examination.

▶ *CourseMate:* Additional practice exercises that further reinforce Chapter 28 content can be found on the CourseMate Web site.

▶ *Recommended minimum time to complete Chapter 28:* 4 to 6 hours, depending on depth of information the instructor wishes to cover and the skill level required by students.

LECTURE OUTLINE CORRELATED TO INSTRUCTOR PRESENTATIONS IN POWERPOINT

The presentations provided contain lecture notes. The notes can be viewed in PowerPoint when viewing the slides in either the normal or outline view. To print the slides with the notes: From your print box look for the "Print What" and change the drop-down to "Notes Pages." A new feature called "Dental Checks" has been interspersed throughout the presentations to keep the student engaged in the materials during the lecture. This feature contains a quick question followed by the answer to stimulate a brief discussion.

1. The Pediatric Dental Office (Slides 2 and 3)

    a. Pediatric Dental Team (Slide 4)

    b. Dental Assistant's Role in Pediatric Dentistry (Slide 5)

2. Behavior Characteristics of Children at Various Ages (Slides 6 and 7)

3. Patient Management (Slides 8 and 9)

    a. Behavioral Assessment

    b. Behavior Management Techniques

        i. Tell, show, and do

        ii. Voice control

        iii. Distraction

        iv. Nonverbal communication

        v. Modeling

        vi. Positive reinforcement

       vii. Gentle restraint

     viii. Hand over mouth

       ix. Mild sedation

        x. General anesthesia

  4. Role of Parent or Guardian (Slide 10)

  5. Procedures in Pediatric Dentistry (Slides 12 through 26)

    a. Examination

    b. Preventive Procedures

       i. Oral hygiene techniques

      ii. Coronal polish

     iii. Pit and fissure sealants

     iv. Fluoride application

      v. Mouth guards

     vi. Orthodontics

    c. Restorative Procedures

       i. Pedodontic matrices

    d. Dental Dam Procedure

    e. Pulp Therapy in Primary and Young Permanent Teeth

    f. Stainless Steel Crowns

  6. Emergency Treatment for Traumatic Injuries (Slides 28 through 33)

    a. Fractured Teeth

    b. Traumatic Intrusion

    c. Displaced Teeth

    d. Avulsed Teeth

  7. Child Abuse (Slides 34 through 37)

    a. The Law and Reporting Child Abuse

Advanced Chairside Functions

  8. Dental Sealants (Slides 38 through 42)

  9. Indications and Contraindications for Sealants

 10. Role of the Dental Assistant

 11. Dental Sealant Materials

12. Bonding, Etching, and Conditioning

13. Placement of Enamel Sealants

TEACHING STRATEGIES

1. Chapter contents are presented in the PowerPoint slides, which are found in the Instructor Resources to Accompany Delmar's *Dental Assisting*.

2. Much of the content in this chapter must be remembered by the student for application in the clinical setting.

3. Students should read the chapter and complete the assignment in *Delmar's Dental Assisting: A Comprehensive Approach Workbook*, followed by hands-on practice to learn pediatric procedures, matrices for children, and placing enamel sealants.

4. Have the students use *Delmar's Dental Assisting Instrument Guide* to assist in their learning of the t-band matrix and the spot-welded matrix.

5. To learn the stages of tooth eruption, have the students examine, using Appendix B in the back of the textbook, several children they know to determine what stage the children are at. Have the students share their findings.

6. Divide the class into groups, have each group research the behavior of a certain age cohort, and then report to whole class ideas that could be used by the dental team to better relate to and understand the specific age group.

7. Invite a pediatric dentist as guest speaker.

CASE STUDY ANSWERS

1. The condition of Noelle's tooth is called "traumatic intrusion."

2. All of Noelle's primary teeth have likely erupted. Traumatic intrusion of the primary teeth may damage the developing permanent teeth.

3. This would be difficult to determine because Noelle is in distress during this visit.

TEXTBOOK REVIEW ANSWERS

Multiple Choice

1. a	2. a	3. b	4. c	5. b	6. b	7. d	8. a
9. c	10. c						

Critical Thinking

1. An office theme or a design that would attract children would include fish or gerbils. In this case, the dental assistant may be responsible for daily feeding and cleaning the tank or cages. A drawing/coloring or toy area may require routine straightening and cleaning.

2. Effective behavior management techniques might include three of the following: tell, show, and do; voice control; distraction; positive nonverbal communication; modeling; and positive reinforcement.

3. Talk with the child about the cuts and bruising. (The injuries may have nothing to do with abuse.) If questions still exist, notify the dentist if you have not already done so, and ask how to proceed. The dentist may wish to ask the parents about the cuts around the face. If the dentist suspects that the child is being abused, he or she may wish to or be obligated to notify a child protection agency so that the situation can be investigated further.

4. Yes, the sealant should be replaced to continue to protect 30 from dental caries. No, the tooth would have to be cleaned and then etched before the sealant is placed.

5. There are several methods to keep the area dry when placing sealants; it is important to find one that works for you. The methods include placing a dental dam, placing cotton rolls and holding them with the fingers, and placing Garmer cotton roll holders.

Periodontics and Coronal Polish

SPECIFIC INSTRUCTIONAL OBJECTIVES

1. Describe the scope of periodontics.

2. Identify members of the periodontal team and their roles.

3. Describe the stages of periodontal disease.

4. Explain the diagnostic procedures involved in the patient's first visit to the periodontal office.

5. Identify and describe periodontal instruments and their uses.

6. Describe nonsurgical procedures and the dental assistant's role in each procedure.

7. Explain surgical procedures and dental assisting responsibilities.

8. Explain the purpose of periodontal dressing.

9. Identify the types of periodontal dressings and how they are prepared, placed, and removed.

10. Describe periodontal maintenance procedures and the patient's role relating to each.

Advanced Chairside Functions

11. Define coronal polish.

12. Describe and explain the rationale for each step in the coronal polish procedure.

13. Explain the indications and contraindications for coronal polish.

14. Describe and identify dental deposits and stains.

15. List types of abrasives and explain characteristics of each type.

16. List and explain types of equipment and materials used to perform a coronal polish.

17. Explain how to maintain the oral cavity during a coronal polish.

18. List auxiliary polishing aids and explain their functions.

19. Describe the steps in the coronal polish procedure.

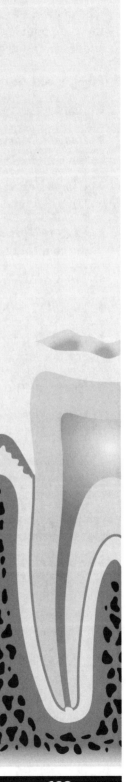

PREPARATORY

Personnel

Primary instructor who is knowledgeable of the dental profession and understands the information the dental assistant needs to know about periodontics as a specialty. This instructor should be a Certified Dental Assistant.

The number of students in a class will determine the number of instructors required for this topic because there are both lecture and clinical portions. In the clinical portion, the student requires hands-on instruction and learning activities that are better accomplished in small groups.

Suggested Audiovisual and Resource Materials

▶ *Workbook:* Chapter 29.

▶ *Image Library:* Provides illustrations from Chapter 29 of the textbook that can be used via computer or as transparencies to provide visual support for classroom instruction.

▶ *Computerized Test Bank:* Provides additional test questions for Chapter 29 and related material on the DANB examination.

▶ *Practice Software:* Additional practice exercises that further reinforce Chapter 29 content can be found on the companion software disk.

▶ *Interactive Skills CD:* Specialty Setups: Periodontics.

▶ *Dental Terminology, Third Edition*: Chapter 16, Periodontics.

▶ *Delmar's Dental Assisting Exam Review:* Additional review material, test questions, and rationales provide practice for the DANB examination.

▶ *Dental Assisting Instrument Guide:* Review of the instrumentation used in periodontic procedures.

▶ *CourseMate:* Additional practice exercises that further reinforce Chapter 29 content can be found on the CourseMate Web site.

▶ *Recommended minimum time to complete Chapter 29:* 4 to 8 hours, depending on depth of information the instructor wishes to cover and the skill level required by students.

LECTURE OUTLINE CORRELATED TO INSTRUCTOR PRESENTATIONS IN POWERPOINT

The presentations provided contain lecture notes. The notes can be viewed in PowerPoint when viewing the slides in either the normal or outline view. To print the slides with the notes: From your print box look for the "Print What" and change the drop-down to "Notes Pages." A new feature called "Dental Checks" has been interspersed throughout the presentations to keep the student engaged in the materials during the lecture. This feature contains a quick question followed by the answer to stimulate a brief discussion.

1. Periodontal Team (Slides 2 and 3)

2. Periodontal Disease (Slides 4 and 5)

   a. Symptoms of Periodontal Disease

   b. Causes of Periodontal Disease

      c. Classifications of Periodontal Disease (Slides 6 through 8)

          i. Gingivitis

         ii. Periodontitis

       iii. Necrotizing Ulcerative Gingivitis and Necrotizing Ulcerative Periodontitis

3. Periodontal Diagnostic Procedures (Slide 10)

    a. Medical Dental History

    b. Clinical Examination (Slides 11 through 14)

    c. Periodontal Screening and Recording System (Slide 15)

    d. Radiographic Interpretation (Slide 16)

    e. Presentation of Treatment Plan (Slide 17)

    f. Chemotherapeutic Agents (Slide 18)

4. Periodontal Instruments (Slides 19 through 26)

    a. Instrument Sharpening

    b. Periodontal Probes

    c. Explorers

    d. Curettes

    e. Scalers

    f. Files

    g. Ultrasonic Instruments

    h. Air polishing systems

    i. Periodontal Knives

    j. Interdental Knives

    k. Periotomes

    l. Surgical Scalpel

    m. Electrosurgery

    n. Pocket Marking Pliers

    o. Periosteal Elevators

    p. Periodontal Scissors, Rongeurs, and Forceps

5. Lasers (Slides 27 through 31)

    a. Uses of the Dental Laser

    b. Benefits of Lasers in Dentistry

6. Nonsurgical Periodontal Procedures (Slides 33 through 35)

   a. Occlusal Adjustment

   b. Scaling and Polishing

   c. Root Planing

   d. Gingival Curettage

   e. Postoperative Treatment

7. Surgical Periodontal Procedures (Slides 37 through 42)

   a. Preoperative Instructions

   b. Gingivectomy

   c. Gingivoplasty

   d. Periodontal Flap Surgery

   e. Osseous Surgery

   f. Mucogingival Surgery

   g. Gingival Grafting

   h. Frenectomy

   i. Guided Tissue Regeneration (GTR)

8. Periodontal Dressing (Slide 43)

   a. Types of Periodontal Dressings

9. Periodontal Maintenance Procedures (Slide 44)

Advanced Chairside Functions (Slides 45 through 47)

10. Coronal Polish

11. Rationale for Performing Coronal Polish

12. Contraindications and Modifications

13. Dental Deposits (Slides 48 through 50)

    a. Soft Deposits

    b. Calculus

    c. Stains

14. Abrasives and Polishing Agents (Slide 51)

    a. Abrasives

    b. Types of Abrasives

15. Equipment and Supplies (Slide 52)

    a. Use of Dental Handpiece for Coronal Polish

    b. Use of the Rubber Prophy Cup

    c. Systematic Procedure

    d. Prophy Brush

    e. Dental Tape and Dental Floss

16. Maintaining Operating Field (Slide 53)

    a. Dental Assistant Guidelines

    b. Patient Considerations

    c. Dental Light Use

    d. Oral Cavity Maintenance

17. Auxiliary Polishing Aids (Slide 54)

    a. Bridge Threaders

    b. Abrasive Polishing Strips

    c. Soft Wood Points

    d. Interproximal Brushes

TEACHING STRATEGIES

1. Chapter contents are presented in the PowerPoint slides, which are found in the Instructor Resources to Accompany Delmar's *Dental Assisting*.

2. Much of the content in this chapter must be remembered by the student for application in the clinical setting.

3. Students should read the chapter and complete the assignment in the workbook followed by hands-on practice to learn the periodontal instruments and procedures and the coronal polish techniques.

4. Have the students use *Delmar's Dental Assisting Instrument Guide* to assist in learning the periodontic instruments.

5. Invite a periodontist as a guest speaker.

CASE STUDY ANSWERS

1. No, Melissa's periodontal readings are not within normal range, which are 1 to 3 in a healthy mouth.

2. Melissa should be asked about the medication she has been taking and other possible precipitating factors in her life.

3. Stress could lead to Melissa grinding her teeth (bruxism) which puts pressure on the teeth and surrounding tissues. Also when a person is under stress their diet may not be healthy and they might not follow good oral hygiene routines.

TEXTBOOK REVIEW ANSWERS

Multiple Choice

1. c   2. b   3. d   4. b   5. c   6. b   7. c   8. b

9. c   10. d

Critical Thinking

1. Bleeding gums, loose teeth, inflammation of the gingiva, periodontal pockets, tenderness, and areas of recession are the signs and symptoms of periodontal disease.

2. Acute necrotizing ulcerative gingivitis (ANUG), also known as Vincent's disease and trench mouth.

3. The dental assistant can provide oral hygiene instructions specific to the needs of the patient; inform the patient about periodontal disease through pamphlets, videos, and models; and encourage and motivate the patient with reminders and phone calls.

4. To keep the fixed bridge clean, a bridge threader could be used to carry the floss under the bridge to keep the area clean and free from debris. In addition, interproximal brushes are flexible and come in different shapes to clean around the abutment teeth of a fixed bridge.

5. Using a fulcrum in some areas takes practice and time to feel comfortable. The ring finger is typically used as the fulcrum finger, but you can try the middle finger and the little finger in some areas. The finger that works the best depends on the size of the operator's hand and the patient's mouth. Although it is ideal to fulcrum on a tooth near the area of operation, sometimes you will need to fulcrum on the soft tissues or on the opposite arch if nothing else feels secure. Practice and try new positions until the fulcrum is comfortable, automatic, and secure.

Fixed Prosthodontics and Gingival Retraction

1. Define the scope of fixed prosthodontics.

2. Explain the dentist's considerations when recommending various prostheses to a patient.

3. Describe various types of fixed prostheses and their functions.

4. Describe dental materials used in fixed prostheses.

5. Identify and explain the CAD/CAM restorative system.

6. Explain the involvement of the laboratory technician in the fabrication of fixed prostheses.

7. Describe the role of the dental assistant in all phases of fixed prosthodontic treatment.

8. Explain techniques for retaining the prosthesis when there is little or no crown on the tooth.

9. Describe implant retainer prostheses.

10. Explain techniques for maintaining fixed prostheses.

Advanced Chairside Function

11. Explain the function of gingival retraction.

12. Describe the different types of gingival retraction.

13. Explain the steps of placing and removing a gingival retraction cord.

PREPARATORY

Personnel

Primary instructor who is knowledgeable of the dental profession and understands what the dental assistant needs to know about fixed prosthodontics as a specialty and the respective procedures completed in the general dental office. This instructor should be a Certified Dental Assistant.

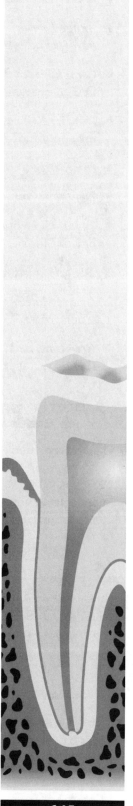

The number of students in a class will determine the number of instructors required for this topic because there are both lecture and clinical portions. In the clinical portion, the student requires hands-on instruction and learning activities that are better accomplished in small groups.

Suggested Audiovisual and Resource Materials

▶ *Workbook:* Chapter 30.

▶ *Image Library:* Provides illustrations from Chapter 30 of the textbook that can be used via computer or as transparencies to provide visual support for classroom instruction.

▶ *Computerized Test Bank:* Provides additional test questions for Chapter 30 and related material on the DANB examination.

▶ *Practice Software:* Additional practice exercises that further reinforce Chapter 30 content can be found on the companion software disk.

▶ *Interactive Skills CD:* Specialty Setups: Prosthodontics.

▶ *Dental Terminology, Third Edition:* Chapter 10, Tooth Restorations; Chapter 12, Prosthodontics.

▶ *Delmar's Dental Assisting Exam Review:* Additional review material, test questions, and rationales provide practice for the DANB examination.

▶ *Dental Assisting Instrument Guide:* Review of the instrumentation used in prosthodontics.

▶ *CourseMate:* Additional practice exercises that further reinforce Chapter 30 content can be found on the CourseMate Web site.

▶ *Recommended minimum time to complete Chapter 30:* 4 to 5 hours, depending on depth of information the instructor wishes to cover and the skill level required by students.

LECTURE OUTLINE CORRELATED TO INSTRUCTOR PRESENTATIONS IN POWERPOINT

The presentations provided contain lecture notes. The notes can be viewed in PowerPoint when viewing the slides in either the normal or outline view. To print the slides with the notes: From your print box look for the "Print What" and change the drop-down to "Notes Pages." A new feature called "Dental Checks" has been interspersed throughout the presentations to keep the student engaged in the materials during the lecture. This feature contains a quick question followed by the answer to stimulate a brief discussion.

1. Role of Dental Assistant (Slides 5 and 6)

2. Patient Considerations (Slides 7 through 10)

   a. Case Presentation

3. Types of Fixed Prostheses (Slides 11 through 22)

   a. Crowns

   b. Inlays and Onlays

   c. Bridges

   d. Veneers

4. Types of Materials Used for Fixed Prostheses (Slides 23 through 26)

   a. Gold Casting Alloys

   b. Tooth-Colored Cast Restorations

5. CAD/CAM Restorative System (Slides 27 through 31)

6. Role of Laboratory Technician (Slides 32 and 33)

7. Fabrication of Prosthesis in Dental Laboratory (Slides 34 and 35)

8. Retention Techniques (Slides 36 through 42)

   a. Core Buildups

   b. Retention Pins

   c. Post-Retained Cores

9. Implant Retainer Prostheses (Slide 43)

10. Maintenance of Fixed Prosthodontics (Slide 44)

    a. Fixed Prostheses Maintenance

    b. Dental Implant Maintenance

11. Crown Preparation Appointment (Slide 45 through 48)

12. Bite Registration (Slides 49 through 54)

13. Try-In Appointment (Slides 55 and 56)

Advanced Chairside Functions (Slides 45 through 51)

14. Gingival Retraction

15. Types of Gingival Retraction

    a. Mechanical Retraction

    b. Retraction Systems

    c. Chemical Retraction

    d. Surgical Retraction

TEACHING STRATEGIES

1. Chapter contents are presented in the PowerPoint slides, which are found in the Instructor Resources to Accompany Delmar's *Dental Assisting*.

2. Much of the content in this chapter must be remembered by the student for application in the clinical setting.

3. Students should read the chapter and complete the assignment in the workbook, followed by hands-on practice to learn the fixed prosthodontic procedures and retraction cord placement.

4. Take the class on a field trip to visit a dental laboratory to see how crowns and bridges are fabricated, and how important it is for the dental lab and the dental office to have good communications.

5. Invite a prosthodontist specialized in fixed appliances as a guest speaker.

CASE STUDY ANSWERS

1. The two concerns that Ann has about her anterior teeth are their appearance and the diastema between the maxillary central incisors.

2. The options for treating the appearance and spacing of the anterior teeth are crowns or veneers.

3. The office manager will explain to the patient whether her insurance covers any part of the treatment.

TEXTBOOK REVIEW ANSWERS

Multiple Choice

1. b   2. b   3. d   4. a   5. c   6. a   7. c   8. b

9. b   10. a

Critical Thinking

1. This varies by state, but could include taking irreversible hydrocolloid impressions (alginate), placing retraction cord, and fabricating and placing temporaries (provisionals).

2. The types of restorations that are fabricated of gold alloy, porcelain fused to metal, or porcelain are crowns, partial crowns, three-quarter crowns, onlays, and inlays.

3. Retentive pins, core buildup, or post-retained cores may be used.

4. If the retraction cord is placed too deep in the sulcus, the crevice opens at the bottom, but is narrow at the top. The dentist may be able to get the impression material into the crevice after the cord is removed, but the material has a tendency to fracture near the edge of the preparation.

5. The dentist may pack two cords to better retract the gingival tissues and thus to increase the crevice opening.

Cosmetic Dentistry and Teeth Whitening

SPECIFIC INSTRUCTIONAL OBJECTIVES

1. Define cosmetic dentistry and describe what is involved in cosmetic dentistry.

2. Describe who performs cosmetic dentistry and education requirements.

3. Explain the role of the dental assistant in cosmetic dentistry.

4. Explain the scope of cosmetic dentistry.

5. Describe fundamental principles that the cosmetic dentist must learn when creating the perfect smile.

6. Discuss the basic elements of psychology and sociology that are considered for cosmetic treatment.

7. Explain what the patient should consider when selecting a dentist for cosmetic treatment.

8. Identify and describe specific procedures performed in cosmetic dentistry, including diagnosis and treatment planning, legal forms, and documentation.

9. Describe the role that oral photography has in cosmetic dentistry, the equipment needed, and how the patient is set up for the photographs to be taken.

10. Describe why soft tissue surgery may be needed in cosmetic dentistry, how it is performed, and how lasers and electrosurgery are involved.

11. Explain why the dental team needs to know about occlusion in cosmetic dentistry.

12. Describe the types of restorations that are placed and materials used for cosmetic restorations.

13. Describe the marketing techniques for cosmetic dentistry.

Advanced Chairside Functions

14. Explain how teeth are whitened, and causes of intrinsic and extrinsic tooth staining.

15. Explain the benefits of whitening techniques used in dentistry.

16. Describe the role of the dental assistant in the whitening process.

17. List and describe types of whitening techniques.

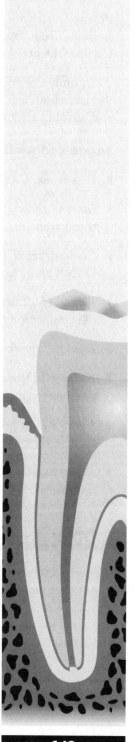

18. Describe the procedures for dental office whitening for vital and nonvital teeth, and for home whitening and over-the-counter whitening materials.

19. Explain information given to the patient about outcomes, procedures, responsibilities, and precautions related to teeth whitening.

PREPARATORY

Personnel

Primary instructor who is knowledgeable of the dental profession and understands the information the dental assistant needs to know about cosmetic dentistry and whitening techniques. This instructor should be a Certified Dental Assistant.

The number of students in a class will determine the number of instructors required for this topic because there are both lecture and clinical portions. In the clinical portion, the student requires hands-on instruction and learning activities that are better accomplished in small groups.

Suggested Audiovisual and Resource Materials

▶ *Workbook:* Chapter 31.

▶ *Image Library:* Provides illustrations from Chapter 31 of the textbook that can be used via computer or as transparencies to provide visual support for classroom instruction.

▶ *Computerized Test Bank:* Provides additional test questions for Chapter 31 and related material on the DANB examination.

▶ *Practice Software:* Additional practice exercises that further reinforce Chapter 31 content can be found on the companion software disk.

▶ *Dental Terminology, Third Edition:* Chapter 11: Cosmetic Dentistry.

▶ *Delmar's Dental Assisting Exam Review:* Additional review material, test questions, and rationales provide practice for the DANB examination.

▶ *CourseMate:* Additional practice exercises that further reinforce Chapter 31 content can be found on the CourseMate Web site.

▶ *Recommended minimum time to complete Chapter 31:* 5 to 8 hours, depending on depth of information the instructor wishes to cover and the skill level required by students.

LECTURE OUTLINE CORRELATED TO INSTRUCTOR PRESENTATIONS IN POWERPOINT

The presentations provided contain lecture notes. The notes can be viewed in PowerPoint when viewing the slides in either the normal or outline view. To print the slides with the notes: From your print box look for the "Print What" and change the drop-down to "Notes Pages." A new feature called "Dental Checks" has been interspersed throughout the presentations to keep the student engaged in the materials during the lecture. This feature contains a quick question followed by the answer to stimulate a brief discussion.

1. Cosmetic Dentist and Staff (Slide 2)

   a. Dental Staff

2. Scope of Cosmetic/Esthetic Dentistry (Slide 3)

3. Fundamentals of Cosmetic Dentistry (Slide 4)

    a. Light

    b. Color

    c. Illusion

    d. Shape and Form

4. Cosmetic Dentistry and Psychology (Slide 6)

    a. Psychological Influences

    b. Sociological Influences

5. How a Patient Selects a Cosmetic Dentist (Slide 7)

6. Procedures in Cosmetic Dentistry (Slide 8)

    a. Diagnosis and Treatment Planning

    b. Legal Forms and Documentation

7. Oral Photography (Slides 9 through 11)

    a. Uses of Oral Photography

    b. Basic Equipment for Dental Photography

    c. Extraoral Techniques

    d. Intraoral Techniques

8. Contouring Soft Tissues in Cosmetic Dentistry (Slide 12)

    a. Indications for Treatment

    b. Methods for Soft Tissue Contouring

    c. Basic Clinic Technique for Soft Tissue Contouring

9. Occlusion in Cosmetic Dentistry (Slide 14)

10. Types of Restorations and Materials (Slides 15 and 16)

11. Marketing Cosmetic Dentistry (Slide 17)

    a. Marketing Plan for the Dental Office

Advanced Chairside Functions

12. Introduction to Tooth Whitening (Slides 18 and 19)

13. Teeth Whitening Shade Guide (Slide 20)

14. How Teeth Are Whitened (Slide 21)

    a. Hydrogen Peroxide

    b. Carbamide Peroxide

    c. Sodium Perborate

15. Causes of Tooth Stains (Slide 22)

16. Role of the Dental Assistant (Slide 23)

17. Whitening Techniques (Slide 24)

    a. Nonvital Whitening

    b. Vital Whitening in Dental Office

    c. Home Whitening Techniques

18. Over-the-Counter Whitening Materials (Slide 25)

    a. Whitening Strips

    b. Whitening Gel

    c. Home Tray Whitening Systems

    d. Whitening Toothpastes

    e. Mouth Rinses and Chewing Gum

19. Patient Information

TEACHING STRATEGIES

1. Chapter contents are presented in the PowerPoint slides, which are found in the Instructor Resources to Accompany Delmar's *Dental Assisting*.

2. Much of the content in this chapter must be remembered by the student for application in the clinical setting.

3. Students should read the chapter and complete the assignment in the workbook, followed by hands-on practice to learn the cosmetic dentistry and whitening procedures.

4. Invite a cosmetic dentist as a guest speaker to the class.

5. Have the students research the Web sites listed at the end of the chapter to learn more about the philosophy, training, and procedures involved in cosmetic dentistry.

6. Design a student project on cosmetic dentistry and then present the information to the class. Each student could be assigned a different aspect of cosmetic dentistry.

7. Organize the students into groups and assign them specific whitening agents and techniques to learn about and then share the information in class.

CASE STUDY ANSWERS

1. Potential problems include tooth sensitivity, gingival tissue irritation, and sloughing of tissue.

2. The dental assistant needs to explain the side effects of tooth whitening and that the patient needs to call the office if any of these symptoms occur. They should be warned to discontinue treatment in the event of tooth sensitivity or tissue irritation.

3. Chance can still have the white teeth he wants. He may have to try one or all of the following suggestions: use a different whitening product, reduce the strength of the whitening solution, or reduce the length of time the bleaching trays are in place. There are many techniques to lighten teeth color; the patient needs to find one that will work for her or him. The dentist and staff are great resources and should always be involved in whatever treatment the patient uses.

TEXTBOOK REVIEW ANSWERS

Multiple Choice

1. c	2. c	3. a	4. d	5. b	6. a	7. d	8. b
9. c	10. a						

Critical Thinking

1. Medical/dental history, two or more study models (one to show existing conditions and one for a mock-up of what the teeth would look like), full mouth set of x-rays, panoramic x-ray, periodontal charting, chart of restorations present, occlusion analysis, and photographs of the patient's face and teeth.

2. It is very important for the dentist to ensure that the patient knows what is involved in the treatment, how much time it will take, and how much the treatment will cost. All of this should be discussed in detail before treatment is started. Cosmetic dentistry is sometimes a compromise between what the patient wants and what the dentist can do, because the two do not always match.

3. Following office policy, the dental assistant could tell the patient about in-office whitening procedures and the importance of consulting with the dentist about his or her specific situation, which technique may be best, and the likely appearance of the outcome.

Removable Prosthodontics

SPECIFIC INSTRUCTIONAL OBJECTIVES

1. Define removable prostheses and list the reasons for using them.

2. Describe considerations about the patient related to removable prosthetic treatment.

3. Explain the dental assistant's role in removable prosthetic treatment.

4. Outline steps of the diagnostic appointment and list the materials needed.

5. Describe the consultation appointment and materials required for the case presentation.

6. Describe advantages and disadvantages of the partial denture, its components, and the appointment schedule.

7. Describe the complete denture, considerations about the patient, and the appointment schedule.

8. Explain the types and steps of denture reline procedures.

9. Describe the procedure for a denture repair.

10. List steps to polish a removable prosthetic appliance.

11. Explain the overdenture and the advantages and disadvantages related to it.

PREPARATORY

Personnel

Primary instructor who is knowledgeable of the dental profession and understands the information the dental assistant needs to know about removable prosthodontics as a specialty and the procedures completed in the general dental office. This instructor should be a Certified Dental Assistant.

The number of students in a class will determine the number of instructors required for this topic because there are both lecture and clinical portions. In the clinical portion, the student requires hands-on instruction and learning activities that are better accomplished in small groups.

Suggested Audiovisual and Resource Materials

▶ *Workbook:* Chapter 32.

▶ *Image Library:* Provides illustrations from Chapter 32 of the textbook that can be used via computer or as transparencies to provide visual support for classroom instruction.

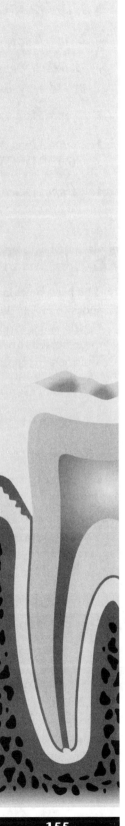

▸ *Computerized Test Bank:* Provides additional test questions for Chapter 32 and related material on the DANB examination.

▸ *Practice Software:* Additional practice exercises that further reinforce Chapter 32 content can be found on the companion software disk.

▸ *Interactive Skills CD:* Specialty Setups: Prosthodontics.

▸ *Dental Terminology, Third Edition:* Chapter 12, Prosthodontics.

▸ *Delmar's Dental Assisting Exam Review:* Additional review material, test questions, and rationales provide practice for the DANB examination.

▸ *Dental Assisting Instruments Guide:* Review of instrumentation used in prosthodontics.

▸ *CourseMate:* Additional practice exercises that further reinforce Chapter 32 content can be found on the CourseMate Web site.

▸ *Recommended minimum time to complete Chapter 32:* 4 to 5 hours, depending on depth of information the instructor wishes to cover and the skill level required by students.

LECTURE OUTLINE CORRELATED TO INSTRUCTOR PRESENTATIONS IN POWERPOINT

The presentations provided contain lecture notes. The notes can be viewed in PowerPoint when viewing the slides in either the normal or outline view. To print the slides with the notes: From your print box look for the "Print What" and change the drop-down to "Notes Pages." A new feature called "Dental Checks" has been interspersed throughout the presentations to keep the student engaged in the materials during the lecture. This feature contains a quick question followed by the answer to stimulate a brief discussion.

1. Patient Considerations (Slide 3)

2. Dental Assistant's Role (Slide 4)

3. Diagnosis and Treatment Planning (Slide 5)

4. Consultation Appointment (Slide 6)

5. Removable Partial Denture (Slides 7 through 10)

   a. Advantages of a Removable Partial Denture

   b. Considerations for a Partial Denture

   c. Components of a Removable Partial Denture

      i. Metal framework

      ii. Rests

      iii. Connectors

      iv. Retainer

      v. Denture base

      vi. Artificial teeth

  d. Partial Denture Procedure

      i. Examination

      ii. Consultation

      iii. Final impressions

      iv. Try-in and adjustment

      v. Delivery

      vi. Adjustment

6. Complete Denture (Slides 12 through 16)

  a. Considerations for a Complete Denture

  b. Necessities for Successful Denture Treatment

  c. Components of a Complete Denture

      i. Denture base

      ii. Denture teeth

  d. Immediate Dentures

  e. Examination and Diagnosis Appointments for a Complete Denture

  f. Consultation and Oral Surgery Appointments

  g. Jaw Relationship Appointment

  h. Denture Construction between Appointments

  i. Denture Construction between Appointments—Laboratory Procedures

  j. Try-In Appointment and Denture Delivery Appointment

  k. Denture Construction between Appointments—Final Laboratory Procedures

  l. Denture Adjustment Appointments

7. Denture Reline (Slides 18 and 19)

8. Denture Repair

9. Polishing Removable Prostheses (Slide 20)

10. Overdenture (Slide 21)

  a. Endosseous Implant and Overdenture for Implant

TEACHING STRATEGIES

1. Chapter contents are presented in the PowerPoint slides, which are found in the Instructor Resources to Accompany Delmar's *Dental Assisting*.

2. Much of the content in this chapter must be remembered by the student for application in the clinical setting.

3. Students should read the chapter and complete the assignment in the workbook, followed by hands-on practice to learn the removable prosthodontic procedures.

4. Take the class on a field trip to visit a dental laboratory to see how dentures and partials are fabricated, and how important it is for the dental lab and the dental office to have good communications.

5. Invite a prosthodontist as a guest speaker.

CASE STUDY ANSWERS

1. The denture procedure that would allow Julie to continue to function with her natural teeth while her maxillary denture is fabricated is called an immediate denture.

2. Pamphlets, videos, and models are among the aids available to help the patient understand the treatment.

3. The dental assistant should consider the patient's overall health, attitude, cooperation, and mental and physical capabilities.

TEXTBOOK REVIEW ANSWERS

Multiple Choice

1. c   2. b   3. c   4. b   5. d   6. c   7. a   8. c

9. b   10. d

Critical Thinking

1. Elastomeric impression materials like polysiloxane can be used to take final impression for partial denture.

2. The baseplates and bite rims must be ready for the jaw relationship appointment.

3. A patient with a few remaining strong, healthy teeth would be a good candidate. An overdenture is a denture designed to fit over a few remaining teeth or dental implants. The denture is designed to attach to the remaining teeth for support and stability.

Dental Cements, Bases, Liners, and Bonding Agents

SPECIFIC INSTRUCTIONAL OBJECTIVES

1. Differentiate between dental cements, bases, liners, and bonding agents.

2. List dental standards and organizations responsible for those standards.

3. Explain the role of the dental assistant in preparing materials.

4. List and explain the properties of dental materials.

5. Identify the types of dental cements. Explain their properties, composition, uses, and manipulation.

6. Describe bonding agents and their manipulation.

7. Describe the steps of cavity preparation.

8. Identify cavity preparation terminology.

Advanced Chairside Functions

9. Classify cavity preparations according to relationship with the pulp.

10. Explain options for protecting the pulp with cavity liners, cavity varnish, and cement bases.

11. Describe the purpose of using cavity liners. List types of materials that can be used and explain the placement procedure.

12. Describe the purpose of using cavity varnish and explain the placement procedure.

13. Describe the purpose of using cement bases. List types of materials that can be used and explain the placement procedure.

PREPARATORY

Personnel

Primary instructor who is knowledgeable of the dental profession and understands the information the dental assistant needs to know about cements, bases, liners, and bonding agents used in procedures completed in the general dental office. This instructor should be a Certified Dental Assistant.

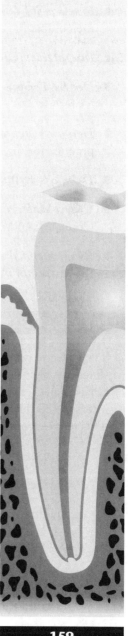

The number of students in a class will determine the number of instructors required for this topic because there are both lecture and clinical portions. In the clinical portion, the student requires hands-on instruction and learning activities that are better accomplished in small groups.

Suggested Audiovisual and Resource Materials

▶ *Workbook:* Chapter 33.

▶ *Delmar's Dental Assisting Video Series:* Appropriate content is available on Tape 4, *Restorative Dental Materials.* This includes mixing glass ionomer, composite restorative materials, dental amalgam, zinc oxide eugenol, and polycarboxylate, as well as assisting with placement of composite restorations.

▶ *Image Library:* Provides illustrations from Chapter 33 of the textbook that can be used via computer or as transparencies to provide visual support for classroom instruction.

▶ *Computerized Test Bank:* Provides additional test questions for Chapter 33 and related material on the DANB examination.

▶ *Practice Software:* Additional practice exercises that further reinforce Chapter 33 content can be found on the companion software disk.

▶ *Interactive Skills CD:* Basic Operative Setups: Amalgam and Composite Trays.

▶ *Dental Terminology, Third Edition:* Chapter 10, Tooth Restorations; Chapter 18, Dental Laboratory Materials.

▶ *Delmar's Dental Assisting Exam Review:* Additional review material, test questions, and rationales provide practice for the DANB examination.

▶ *Delmar's Dental Assisting Materials Guide:* Review materials used in restorative dentistry procedures.

▶ *CourseMate:* Additional practice exercises that further reinforce Chapter 33 content can be found on the CourseMate Web site.

▶ *Recommended minimum time to complete Chapter 33:* 4 to 6 hours, depending on depth of information the instructor wishes to cover and the skill level required by students.

LECTURE OUTLINE CORRELATED TO INSTRUCTOR PRESENTATIONS IN POWERPOINT

The presentations provided contain lecture notes. The notes can be viewed in PowerPoint when viewing the slides in either the normal or outline view. To print the slides with the notes: From your print box look for the "Print What" and change the drop-down to "Notes Pages." A new feature called "Dental Checks" has been interspersed throughout the presentations to keep the student engaged in the materials during the lecture. This feature contains a quick question followed by the answer to stimulate a brief discussion.

1. Role of the Dental Assistant (Slide 4)

2. Properties of Dental Materials (Slides 5 through 8)

    a. Acidity

    b. Adhesion

    c. Biting Forces

    d. Corrosion

    e. Dimensional Change

  f. Elasticity

  g. Flow

  h. Galvanism

  i. Hardness

  j. Microleakage

  k. Retention

  l. Bonding

  m. Solubility

  n. Thermal Properties

  o. Viscosity

  p. Wettability

3. Types of Restorative Dental Materials (Slide 10)

  a. Liners, bases, cements, bonding agents

  b. Amalgam, composite, glass ionomer

4. Dental Cements (Slides 11 through 28)

  a. Uses of Dental Cements

  b. Zinc Phosphate Cement

  c. Zinc Oxide Eugenol Cement

  d. Polycarboxylate Cement

  e. Glass Ionomer Cement

  f. Resin-Modified Glass Ionomer

  g. Calcium Hydroxide Material

  h. Cavity Varnish

  i. Resin Cement

  j. Compomer Cement

  k. Etchants

5. Bonding Agents (Slide 29)

  a. Enamel Bonding

  b. Dentin Bonding

6. Restorative Dentistry (Slides 31 through 33)

  a. Classification

  b. Cavity Detection

    c. Cavity Cleaners/Disinfectants

    d. Desensitizers

    e. Cavity Preparation Identification

    f. Elements of Cavity Preparation

Advanced Chairside Functions

7. Placing Cement, Bases, and Liners (Slide 34)

8. Cavity Preparation/Pulpal Involvement

9. Treatment of Cavity Preparations (Slides 35 through 37)

10. Cavity Liners (Slide 38)

11. Cavity Varnish (Slides 39 and 40)

12. Cement Bases (Slide 41)

TEACHING STRATEGIES

1. Chapter contents are presented in the PowerPoint slides, which are found in the Instructor Resources to Accompany Delmar's *Dental Assisting*.

2. Much of the content in this chapter must be remembered by the student for application in the clinical setting.

3. Students should read the chapter and complete the assignment in the workbook, followed by hands-on practice to learn dental cements, bases, liners, and bonding agents.

4. Show the *Delmar Dental Assisting* video on mixing dental cements, bases, and liners.

5. Invite a dentist and/or a dental sales representative as a guest speaker.

6. Have the students make note cards on each material to assist in learning the various categories and types.

7. Have models available of the different types of restorations and a photo or model of a cavity preparation so that the students can learn when each material is used.

CASE STUDY ANSWERS

1. The steps that can be taken to reduce or eliminate sensitivity problems include the placing of liners and a base to soothe and protect the pulp. Some of these materials contain fluoride that helps to strengthen the tooth structure, which in turn will reduce sensitivity.

2. The dental assistant could explain to the patient the steps the dentist took to reduce or eliminate sensitivity, and that sometimes the tooth is sensitive right after the filling but that the sensitivity should decrease with time.

TEXTBOOK REVIEW ANSWERS

Multiple Choice

1. b   2. d   3. c   4. c   5. a   6. d   7. a   8. d

9. c   10. b

Critical Thinking

1. Two examples of thermal conductivity relating to dentistry would be a patient drinking hot coffee while wearing a denture and a patient with sensitive teeth after chewing ice.

2. Some cements have specific drops and dispensers that are used to obtain a certain consistency. The size of the tooth and restoration may determine the amount of powder and liquid.

3. Cavity varnish would be placed over the calcium hydroxide because the varnish seals the dentin tubules, and calcium hydroxide should be placed near or over the pulp.

Restorative Materials, Dental Dam, Matrix, and Wedge

SPECIFIC INSTRUCTIONAL OBJECTIVES

1. Explain the properties, composition, and manipulation of dental amalgam.

2. Identify the armamentarium and steps of an amalgam procedure.

3. Explain the composition of composite resins.

4. Explain the properties and manipulation of various composite restorations.

5. Identify the armamentarium and steps of a composite restoration.

6. Explain the use of glass ionomer, resin, resin-reinforced glass ionomer, and compomer restorative materials.

Advanced Chairside Functions

7. Explain the purpose of the dental dam and identify who places it on a patient.

8. List and explain advantages and contraindications of the dental dam.

9. Identify the armamentarium needed for the dental dam procedure and explain the function of each.

10. Explain how to prepare the patient for dental dam placement and how to determine the isolation area. Describe and demonstrate how dental dam material is prepared.

11. List and demonstrate steps of placing and removing the dental dam.

12. Explain and demonstrate the dental dam procedure for the child patient.

13. Define matrix and wedge. List the uses and types of matrices.

14. Describe the functions, parts, placement, and removal of the Tofflemire matrix.

15. Explain and demonstrate placement and removal of the strip matrix.

PREPARATORY

Personnel

Primary instructor who is knowledgeable about the dental profession and understands the information the dental assistant needs to know about restorative

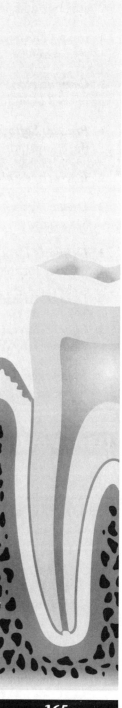

materials, the dental dam, and the matrix and wedge used in procedures completed in the general dental office. This instructor should be a Certified Dental Assistant.

The number of students in a class will determine the number of instructors required for this topic because there are both lecture and clinical portions. In the clinical portion, the student requires hands-on instruction and learning activities that are better accomplished in small groups.

Suggested Audiovisual and Resource Materials

▶ *Workbook:* Chapter 34.

▶ *Delmar's Dental Assisting Video Series:* Appropriate content is available on Tape 4, *Restorative Dental Materials.* This includes mixing glass ionomer, composite restorative materials, dental amalgam, zinc oxide eugenol, and polycarboxylate, as well as assisting with placement of composite restorations.

▶ *Image Library:* Provides illustrations from Chapter 34 of the textbook that can be used via computer or as transparencies to provide visual support for classroom instruction.

▶ *Computerized Test Bank:* Provides additional test questions for Chapter 34 and related material on the DANB examination.

▶ *Practice Software:* Additional practice exercises that further reinforce Chapter 34 content can be found on the companion software disk.

▶ *Interactive Skills CD:* Basic Operative Setups: Amalgam and Composite Trays.

▶ *Dental Terminology, Third Edition:* Chapter 10, Tooth Restorations; Chapter 18, Dental Laboratory Materials.

▶ *Delmar's Dental Assisting Exam Review:* Additional review material, test questions, and rationales provide practice for the DANB examination.

▶ *Dental Assisting Materials Guide:* Review materials used in restorative procedures.

▶ *CourseMate:* Additional practice exercises that further reinforce Chapter 34 content can be found on the CourseMate Web site.

▶ *Recommended minimum time to complete Chapter 34:* 4 to 6 hours, depending on depth of information the instructor wishes to cover and the skill level required by students.

LECTURE OUTLINE CORRELATED TO INSTRUCTOR PRESENTATIONS IN POWERPOINT

The presentations provided contain lecture notes. The notes can be viewed in PowerPoint when viewing the slides in either the normal or outline view. To print the slides with the notes: From your print box look for the "Print What" and change the drop-down to "Notes Pages." A new feature called "Dental Checks" has been interspersed throughout the presentations to keep the student engaged in the materials during the lecture. This feature contains a quick question followed by the answer to stimulate a brief discussion.

1. Amalgam Restorative Materials (Slides 2 and 3)

   a. Composition

   b. Types of Dental Amalgam

   c. Mercury Used in Dental Amalgam

      i. Mercury hygiene program

d. Forms of Dental Alloy

e. Amalgam Properties

    i. Expansion and contraction

    ii. Creep

    iii. Tarnish and corrosion

f. Amalgam Manipulation

g. Amalgam Bonding

h. Complete Amalgam Procedure

2. Composite Restorative Materials (Slide 4)

    a. Composite Composition

        i. Organic polymer matrix

        ii. Inorganic filler particles

        iii. Organic silane coupling agents

        iv. Macrofill, microfill, hybrid

        v. Flowable composites

        vi. Packable composites

    b. Composite Properties

    c. Manipulation Considerations

    d. Modifications

        i. Classes I and II

        ii. Class IV

        iii. Class V

3. Glass Ionomer Restorations (Slide 5)

    a. Hybrid (or Resin-Modified) Glass Ionomers

4. Compomers (Slide 6)

Advanced Chairside Functions

5. Dental Dam (Slides 8 through 18)

    a. Advantages of Dental Dam Use

    b. Contraindication to Dental Dam Isolation

    c. Materials and Equipment

        i. Dental Dam Materials

        ii. Dental Dam Napkin

   iii. Dental Dam Frame

   iv. Dental Dam Punching Guides

   v. Dental Dam Punch

   vi. Dental Dam Clamps

   vii. Dental Dam Forceps

   viii. Dental Floss

   ix. Lubricant

   x. Scissors

   xi. Inverting or Tucking Instrument

   xii. Ligatures

   xiii. Stabilizing Cord

  d. Preparation Before Dental Dam Placement

   i. Educating the Patient

   ii. Determining Area to Isolate

   iii. Dividing the Dental Dam

   iv. Punching the Dental Dam

  e. Common Errors When Punching Dental Dam

  f. Placement and Removal Procedures for Dental Dam

  g. Dental Dam for Pediatric Patients

  h. Placing Dental Dam for Pediatric Patients

6. Alternatives to Full Dental Dam Placement

7. Matrix and Wedge (Slides 20 through 22)

  a. Matrices

  b. Wedges

   i. Wedge Types

   ii. Wedge Placement

  c. Tofflemire Matrix

   i. Parts of Tofflemire Matrix Retainer

   ii. Matrix Bands

  d. AutoMatrix

  e. Plastic Strip Matrix

  f. Sectional Matrix Systems

TEACHING STRATEGIES

1. Chapter contents are presented in the PowerPoint slides, which are found in the Instructor Resources to Accompany Delmar's *Dental Assisting*.

2. Much of the content in this chapter must be remembered by the student for application in the clinical setting.

3. Students should read the chapter and complete the assignment in the workbook, followed by hands-on practice to learn the restorative materials, the dental dam, and the matrix and wedge.

4. Show the *Delmar Dental Assisting* video on restorative materials and the dental dam.

5. Invite a dentist and/or dental sales representative as guest speaker(s).

6. Have the students make note cards on each material to assist in learning the various categories and types.

7. Bring in models of the various types of restorations and a photo or model of a cavity preparation so that the students can learn when each material is used.

8. Demonstrate the various restorative materials and have the students prepare the materials to assist in understanding not only each material's respective composition, characteristics, and properties, but also how they are used in restorative procedures.

9. Demonstrate the dental dam being placed on a patient so that the students can visualize the steps in placing and removing the dental dam.

10. Show the video by the Hygienic Company called *Dam It's Easy*.

CASE STUDY ANSWERS

1. Charlotte may have read about concerns that the level of mercury may be greater in patients with numerous amalgam restorations and concerns that patients may ingest a low amount of mercury from the amalgam restorations. Another concern involves a possible risk of an allergic reaction to mercury.

2. The dental assistant could give information to Charlotte from the American Dental Association that includes current studies and recommendations.

3. Yes, composite restorative materials, glass ionomers, and porcelain would be available to Charlotte as alternatives to amalgam restoration material.

TEXTBOOK REVIEW ANSWERS

Multiple Choice

1. a	2. b	3. b	4. a	5. a	6. d	7. c	8. c
9. d	10. b						

Critical Thinking

1. Pros: low cost, easy to place, long lasting; overall, a dependable and safe restorative material. Cons: aesthetics ranks rather low, and contains mercury, which is somewhat hazardous and needs to be handled properly.

2. The pulp can be protected with a cavity liner before the etching and bonding of the composite.

3. There are several alternatives to composites, including resin-modified glass ionomer and compomers.

4. The advantages for the dental assistant include controlled area when evacuating, better retraction of the tongue and cheeks, and better visibility.

5. Refer to Procedure 34-7.

CHAPTER 35

Laboratory Materials and Techniques

SPECIFIC INSTRUCTIONAL OBJECTIVES

1. Identify materials used in the dental laboratory and perform associated procedures.

2. Demonstrate the knowledge and skills needed to prepare, take, and remove alginate impressions and wax bites.

3. Demonstrate the knowledge and skills necessary to prepare reversible hydrocolloid impression material for the dentist.

4. Demonstrate the knowledge and skills necessary to prepare elastomeric impression materials such as polysulfide, silicone (polysiloxane and polyvinyl siloxanes), and polyether for the dentist.

5. Demonstrate the knowledge and skills necessary to use gypsum products such as Type I, impression plaster; Type II, laboratory or model plaster; Type III, laboratory stone; Type IV, die stone; and Type V, high-strength die stone.

6. Demonstrate the knowledge and skills necessary to pour and trim a patient's alginate impression (diagnostic cast).

7. Identify the use of a dental articulator and facebow for dental casts or study models.

8. Demonstrate taking a facebow transfer and mounting models on an articulator.

9. Identify various classifications and uses of waxes used in dentistry.

10. Demonstrate the knowledge and skills necessary to fabricate acrylic tray resin self-curing and light-curing custom trays, vacuum-formed trays, and thermoplastic custom trays.

11. Demonstrate the knowledge and skills necessary to contour prefabricated temporary crowns and to fabricate and fit custom temporary restorations.

12. Gain an understanding of computer-aided design (CAD) equipment and computer-aided manufacturing (CAM) systems and how they are used in the dental office.

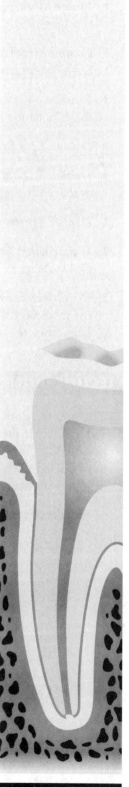

PREPARATORY

Personnel

Primary instructor should have experience as a dental laboratory technician, or have a dental assisting background with time spent performing dental laboratory procedures.

Suggested Audiovisual and Resource Materials

▶ *Workbook:* Chapter 35.

▶ *Delmar's Dental Assisting Video Series:* Appropriate content is available on Tape 5, *Laboratory Impressions, Materials, and Techniques*. This includes taking an alginate impression, trimming casts and study models, and taking a bite registration.

▶ *Image Library:* Provides illustrations from Chapter 35 of the textbook that can be used via computer or as transparencies to provide visual support for classroom instruction.

▶ *Computerized Test Bank:* Provides additional test questions for Chapter 35 and related material on the DANB examination.

▶ *Practice Software:* Additional practice exercises that further reinforce Chapter 35 content can be found on the companion software disk.

▶ *Dental Terminology, Third Edition:* Chapter 18, Dental Laboratory Materials.

▶ *Delmar's Dental Assisting Exam Review:* Additional review material, test questions, and rationales provide practice for the DANB examination.

▶ *Dental Assisting Materials Guide:* Review materials used in laboratory procedures.

▶ *CourseMate:* Additional practice exercises that further reinforce Chapter 35 content can be found on the CourseMate Web site.

▶ *Recommended minimum time to complete Chapter 35:* 8 to 10 hours, depending on depth of information the instructor wishes to cover. This material should also be taught with an additional 10 to 15 hours of laboratory skill development.

LECTURE OUTLINE CORRELATED TO INSTRUCTOR PRESENTATIONS IN POWERPOINT

The presentations provided contain lecture notes. The notes can be viewed in PowerPoint when viewing the slides in either the normal or outline view. To print the slides with the notes: From your print box look for the "Print What" and change the drop-down to "Notes Pages." A new feature called "Dental Checks" has been interspersed throughout the presentations to keep the student engaged in the materials during the lecture. This feature contains a quick question followed by the answer to stimulate a brief discussion.

1. Hydrocolloid Impression Materials (Slides 2 through 9)

    a. Alginate (Irreversible Hydrocolloid) Impression Material

        i. Advantages and disadvantages

        ii. Setting time

        iii. Packaging, storage, and shelf life

        iv. Powder/water ratio

        v. Materials needed

        vi. Trays used

        vii. Study models

2. Wax Bite Registration (Slide 10)

3. Reversible Hydrocolloid Impression Material (Agar-Agar) (Slide 11)

   a. Advantages and disadvantages

   b. Packaging and equipment

4. Elastomeric Impression Materials (Slide 12)

5. Polysulfide (Slides 13 and 14)

6. Silicone (Polysiloxane and Polyvinal Siloxanes) (Slide 15)

7. Polyether (Slide 16)

8. Gypsum Materials (Slides 18 and 19)

   a. Plaster

   b. Type I: Impression Plaster

   c. Type II: Laboratory or Model Plaster

   d. Type III: Laboratory Stone

   e. Orthodontic Stone

   f. Type IV: Die Stone

   g. Type V: High-Strength, High-Expansion Die Stone

   h. Trimming and Finishing Diagnostic Casts

9. Articulating Casts or Study Models (Slide 20)

10. Facebows and Articulators (Slide 21)

    a. Facebow transfer

    b. Articulator

11. Dental Waxes (Slides 22 through 24)

    a. Wax Groups

    b. Pattern Wax

    c. Processing Wax

    d. Impression or Bite Registration Waxes

    e. Additional Waxes

12. Custom Trays (Slide 25)

    a. Acrylic Tray Resin Self-Curing Custom Trays

    b. Acrylic Tray Resin Light-Cured Custom Trays

    c. Vacuum-Formed Custom Trays

    d. Thermoplastic Tray Material Custom Trays

13. Constructing a Custom Tray (Slide 26)

    a. Outlining Tray Margins

14. Vacuum-Formed Tray (Slide 27)

15. Temporary (Provisional) Restorations (Slide 28)

    a. Types of Temporary Restorations

    b. Preformed Aluminum Temporary Crowns

    c. Preformed Acrylic Temporary Crowns

    d. Custom Acrylic or Composite Temporary Restorations

16. CAD/CAM and Digital Impressions (Slide 29)

    a. Digital Impressions

    b. Computer-Aided Design

    c. Computer-Aided Manufacturing

TEACHING STRATEGIES

1. Chapter contents are presented in the PowerPoint slides, which are found in the Instructor Resources to Accompany Delmar's *Dental Assisting*.

2. When learning about dental laboratory materials, it is best that students see the materials and handle them as well. This class is best taught concurrently with a laboratory class in which students can use the materials and complete the skills as shown in the student workbook that corresponds with the main textbook.

3. Many local dental laboratories will allow for student tours, which can be arranged by instructors.

4. Have students deliver a written assignment following a dental laboratory visit. For instance, after the students have observed the manufacture of ceramic crowns, they would then seek additional information on the Web.

5. Many assignments covering the topics in this chapter are possible, such as evaluating gypsum product pouring and taking impressions. This content most often covers a number of skills being completed as noted in the student workbook.

CASE STUDY ANSWER

1. To help Patrick with the gagging reflex problem, the dental assistant can seat the patient upright, have him rinse his mouth, explain the procedure, ensure that the tray fits properly, take the mandibular impression first, and remove a small amount of impression material from the palate area of the maxillary tray prior to placement in the oral cavity.

2. Alginate (irreversible hydrocolloid) impression material is routinely used in obtaining preliminary impressions.

3. Fast set would be most beneficial for a patient with a gag problem because the time in the mouth is reduced.

4. The mandibular arch would be taken first to build confidence, allowing the patient to feel more secure.

TEXTBOOK REVIEW ANSWERS

Multiple Choice

1. b	2. d	3. a	4. c	5. d	6. a	7. b	8. d
9. a	10. d						

Critical Thinking

1. Types of final impression material include reversible hydrocolloid, polysiloxane, polysulfide, polyether, and silicone. Factors affecting their usage include equipment needed to take the impression, time for pouring, stability of material, taste and odor of material, trays needed, cost, and accuracy.

2. The effects of a lower water-to-powder ratio in a mixture of irreversible hydrocolloid include decreased detail, ability to pull from undercuts, and flexibility; increased tissue displacement, setting time, and strength; and a mixture that lacks uniform consistency.

3. Advantages include accuracy, dimensional stability, and rapid setting time in the mouth. Additionally, it comes in several forms, is easy to manipulate and easy to clean up after use, and its odor and taste are well tolerated by the patient.

CHAPTER 36

Dental Office Management

SPECIFIC INSTRUCTIONAL OBJECTIVES

1. Identify the dental office staff and their areas of responsibility.

2. Identify marketing ideas for dentistry.

3. Outline the proper procedure for answering an incoming call.

4. Describe the information every message should contain.

5. Describe telephone and business office technology and its uses.

6. Give examples of the ways in which computers are used in the dental office.

7. Explain how database management concepts can be used in the dental office.

8. Explain why ergonomics is important at a computer workstation.

9. Explain ways in which effective patient scheduling can be accomplished in the dental office.

10. Identify the equipment needed for record management.

11. Define key terms related to accounts receivable.

12. Identify computerized and manual systems for management of patient accounts.

13. Identify accounts payable expenses that the dental practice is responsible for.

PREPARATORY

Personnel

Instructors should have a background in dental assisting and have had experience working in the front office. An instructor who has worked as office manager or receptionist in a dental office would also be beneficial.

Suggested Audiovisual and Resource Materials

▶ *Workbook:* Chapter 36.

▶ *Image Library:* Provides illustrations from Chapter 36 of the textbook that can be used via computer or as transparencies to provide visual support for classroom instruction.

▶ *Computerized Test Bank:* Provides additional test questions for Chapter 36 and related material on the DANB examination.

▶ *Practice Software:* Additional practice exercises that further reinforce Chapter 36 content can be found on the companion software disk.

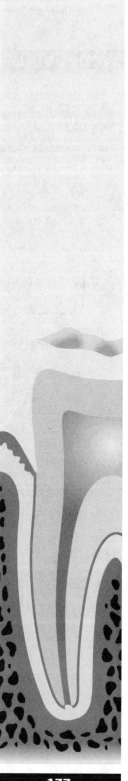

177

▶ *Dental Terminology, Third Edition:* Chapter 20, Business Procedures.

▶ *Delmar's Dental Assisting Exam Review:* Additional review material, test questions, and rationales provide practice for the DANB examination.

▶ *CourseMate:* Additional practice exercises that further reinforce Chapter 36 content can be found on the CourseMate Web site.

▶ *Recommended minimum time to complete Chapter 36:* 8 to 10 hours, depending on depth of information the instructor wishes to cover and the videos available to the instructor.

LECTURE OUTLINE CORRELATED TO INSTRUCTOR PRESENTATIONS IN POWERPOINT

The presentations provided contain lecture notes. The notes can be viewed in PowerPoint when viewing the slides in either the normal or outline view. To print the slides with the notes: From your print box look for the "Print What" and change the drop-down to "Notes Pages." A new feature called "Dental Checks" has been interspersed throughout the presentations to keep the student engaged in the materials during the lecture. This feature contains a quick question followed by the answer to stimulate a brief discussion.

1. Reception Area (Slide 2)

2. Dental Receptionist and Business Office Staff (Slides 3 through 6)

   a. Dental Receptionist

   b. Dental Office Bookkeeper

3. Dentistry Marketing (Slides 7 and 8)

4. U.S. Postal Service (Slides 9 and 10)

   a. USPS Services

5. Telephone Technique (Slides 11 through 13)

   a. Basic Telephone Techniques

   b. Call Types

   c. Answering Calls

   d. Placing Callers on Hold

   e. Taking Messages

   f. Outgoing Calls

   g. Long-Distance Calls

   h. English as a Second Language

   i. Telephone and Business Office Technology

6. Business Office Systems (Slide 15)

   a. Common Dental Office Software

   b. Database Management

   c. Computer Safety

7. Patient Scheduling (Slide 16)

   a. Appointment Books

   b. Computer Scheduling

   c. Appointment Book Entries

   d. Recall Patients

8. Dental Records Management (Slides 17 and 18)

   a. Equipment and Supplies for Record Management

   b. Patient Chart Filing

   c. Record Confidentiality

   d. Mandated Electronic Recordkeeping by 2014

   e. Daily Schedule

9. Accounts Receivable (Slide 19)

   a. Patient Fees

10. Patient Account Management (Slides 22 and 23)

   a. Pegboard System of Account Management

   b. Computer System of Account Management

   c. Monthly Billing

   d. Financial Information

   e. Dental Insurance

   f. Capitation Program

   g. Contract Fee Schedule Plan

   h. Direct Reimbursement Plans

   i. Managed Care Plans

   j. Submitting Dental Insurance Claims

   k. Dental Service Payment

   l. Collection Management

   m. Special Collection Situations

   n. Recording Payments

11. Accounts Payable (Slides 24 through 27)

    a. Inventory Supply Systems

    b. Account Payment

    c. Petty Cash

    d. Payroll

12. Staying Current

    a. Trends

    b. Seminars

    c. Mobile services

    d. Web conferencing

TEACHING STRATEGIES

1. Chapter contents are presented in the PowerPoint slides, which are found in the Instructor Resources to Accompany Delmar's *Dental Assisting*.

2. Many videos on accounting procedures are available. Even more important than such procedures per se are patient, team member, and dentist interactions. Numerous videos or DVDs showing interpersonal communication in the health care industry can be obtained from school libraries or public libraries.

3. When students learn about dental office management, they should obtain a comprehensive view of the skills that the dental front office personnel provide. A number of packets are available that provide the steps to manage an office and the accounting skills to be developed. Students should complete such packets on their own or in the classroom to ensure that all areas are covered. The packets normally have students work with developing a chart, patient continuing care (recall), accounts receivable and payable, inventory control, payroll, and filing. Each segment is completed in a progressive manner to provide students with a basic understanding of office management. The packet can be assigned along with tasks from the textbook.

4. Spending time in the business/reception areas of a dental office to evaluate skills used in efficient office management would be beneficial for all students.

5. Have students interview a dental office manager about necessary job skills and what they would look for in hiring people to work in their office.

6. All students should obtain training on a dental software program to perform many of the skills routinely used in the dental office business/reception areas.

CASE STUDY ANSWERS

1. Word processing for memos, letters, and reports; graphics; spreadsheets; welcoming letters, birthday cards, and thank-you notes for marketing purposes; and management functions can be performed on a computer-based dental practice management system.

2. Monthly and yearly financial reports, accounts payable and receivable, and production reports can be generated.

3. In her educational program, Melissa should have studied practice management.

TEXTBOOK REVIEW ANSWERS

Multiple Choice

1. d　　2. b　　3. d　　4. c　　5. a　　6. b　　7. c　　8. d

9. b　　10. a

Critical Thinking

1. The practice is a business, and it must collect accounts receivable to enable it to provide quality service to patients. In a successful practice, collections are performed promptly and accurately.

2. Section one—record of charges and receipts; section two—record of deposits; section three—business analysis record; section four—record of where balances are totaled; section five—proof of posting and accounts receivable control.

3. Color-coding makes chart retrieval and filing more efficient.

Employment Strategies

SPECIFIC INSTRUCTIONAL OBJECTIVES

1. Identify three pathways to obtain DANB certification.

2. Explain how to obtain employment and identify types of practices.

3. Set goals and identify sources to obtain employment in the dental field.

4. Identify the steps in preparing a cover letter and résumé.

5. Define how to prepare for the interview.

6. Explain the interview process and identify skills and preparation techniques that will aid in obtaining the job.

7. Identify the skills that a successful dental assistant possesses.

8. Explain how to terminate employment.

PREPARATORY

Personnel

Instructors should be certified by the Dental Assisting National Board and understand employment in the area and across the nation for dental assistants.

Suggested Audiovisual and Resource Materials

▶ *Workbook:* Chapter 37.

▶ *Image Library:* Provides illustrations from Chapter 37 of the textbook that can be used via computer or as transparencies to provide visual support for classroom instruction.

▶ *Computerized Test Bank:* Provides additional test questions for Chapter 37 and related material on the DANB examination.

▶ *Practice Software:* Additional practice exercises that further reinforce Chapter 37 content can be found on the companion software disk.

▶ *Dental Terminology, Third Edition:* Chapter 20, Business Management Procedures.

▶ *Delmar's Dental Assisting Exam Review:* Additional review material, test questions, and rationales provide practice for the DANB examination.

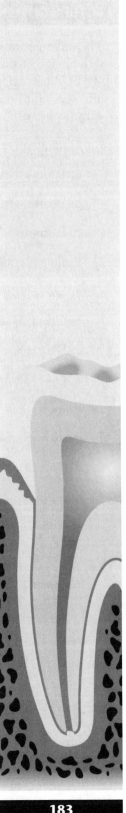

◗ *CourseMate:* Additional practice exercises that further reinforce Chapter 37 content can be found on the CourseMate Web site.

◗ *Recommended minimum time to complete Chapter 37:* 3 to 4 hours, depending on depth of information the instructor wishes to cover and videos available to instructor.

LECTURE OUTLINE CORRELATED TO INSTRUCTOR PRESENTATIONS IN POWERPOINT

The presentations provided contain lecture notes. The notes can be viewed in PowerPoint when viewing the slides in either the normal or outline view. To print the slides with the notes: From your print box look for the "Print What" and change the drop-down to "Notes Pages." A new feature called "Dental Checks" has been interspersed throughout the presentations to keep the student engaged in the materials during the lecture. This feature contains a quick question followed by the answer to stimulate a brief discussion.

1. Obtaining National Certification (Slide 2)

   a. Pathway I

   b. Pathway II

   c. Pathway III

2. Employment (Slides 7 and 8)

   a. Solo or Partnership Practice

   b. Group Practice

   c. Dental Specialty Practice

   d. Other Employment Choices

3. Employment Search (Slides 9 and 10)

4. Preparing a Cover Letter and Résumé (Slides 11 through 13)

   a. Cover Letter

   b. Résumé

5. Setting Up an Interview

6. Interview Process (Slide 14)

   a. Leaving Interview and Following Up

   b. Receiving an Employment Offer

7. Professional Conduct During Employment (Slides 15 and 16)

   a. Terminating Employment

   b. Continued Success

TEACHING STRATEGIES

1. Chapter contents are presented in the PowerPoint slides, which are found in the Instructor Resources to Accompany Delmar's *Dental Assisting*.

2. Several videos are available that show how to prepare for and behave during an interview for employment. Most school libraries have such DVDs or videos.

3. Many software packages are available to aid students in preparing a cover letter and résumé. The textbook discusses cover letter essentials. Students should prepare a résumé and cover letter upon completion of this chapter.

4. Role-playing employment interviews is useful, particularly when the interviewers are people with experience in hiring personnel. Such interviewers can provide invaluable feedback to students.

5. Have students seek the application for the Dental Assisting National Board examination, complete the examination, and turn it in for evaluation.

CASE STUDY ANSWERS

1. Svetlana should bring her portfolio with letters of recommendation, copies of certificates, and radiographs she has taken or any additional items that will attest to her ability and skills. She should have a current cover letter, a résumé, and a list of questions that can be asked of the dentist and staff.

2. Svetlana can practice by asking a friend or family member to do a mock interview and provide feedback on areas that can be improved.

3. She should wear something comfortable, dress appropriately, and demonstrate good hygiene. Clothes must be clean, pressed, and aimed at a conservative and professional presentation.

4. Svetlana should allow additional time to get to the interview and be 5 to 10 minutes early to prepare for the interview process.

TEXTBOOK REVIEW ANSWERS

Multiple Choice

1. c	2. d	3. b	4. a	5. d	6. b	7. d	8. b
9. b	10. d						

Critical Thinking

1. Talk to current employees of the dentist, identify the office philosophy, and identify the type of dental practice.

2. A solo practice comprises one dentist, a partnership two dentists, and a group practice several independent dentists. In a dental specialty practice, only treatments within a given specialty are offered.

3. A dental assistant may obtain employment in private and specialty dental practices, government clinics, dental and dental assisting schools, veterans' hospitals, dental supply companies, and insurance companies.

Using Dental Practice Management Software

The student workbook contains a DENTRIX® G4 Learning CD that will assist your students in mastering dental software skills. Working with DENTRIX® allows students to build a technology foundation that can be transferred to other dental management systems.

Because of the wide range of student competencies in using technology, Part II of the workbook is designed to be "self-paced" by the student with guidance by an instructor. Part II covers Patient Management skills first and Practice Management skills second. Instructors have the option of using both parts of Part II simultaneously or using the parts separately. To be successful with the Patient Management section, it should be taught after completion of Section 4, Chapter 16 of the textbook and workbook. The Practice Management skills should be taught after the completion of Chapter 37 so students begin with a background in office management.

Patient Management

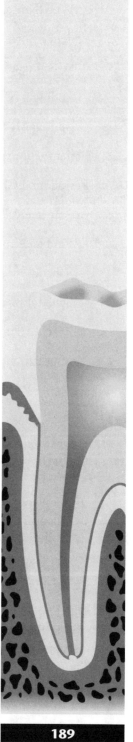

SPECIFIC INSTRUCTIONAL OBJECTIVES

1. Using the Internet, identify at least two practice management software programs in addition to DENTRIX®.

2. Discuss three reasons the clinical dental team should be able to create and edit a patient chart.

3. Using DENTRIX®, demonstrate retrieving patient information with different search methods.

4. Explain why multiple search methods would be beneficial.

5. Demonstrate entering a family group into DENTRIX®.

6. Demonstrate how to add charting for a patient in the DENTRIX® sample practice database.

7. Demonstrate how to add periodontal charting for a patient in the DENTRIX® sample practice database.

8. Using DENTRIX®, demonstrate adding a photo to an existing patient's chart.

9. Using DENTRIX®, create an appointment for a new patient and an existing patient; then demonstrate moving those appointments to other days and times.

PREPARATORY

Personnel

It would be helpful for the instructor providing guidance for practice management software to have a working knowledge of dental software. This does not have to be DENTRIX®. Because Part I does contain charting (both dental and periodontal), prescriptions, and noting medical alerts, an instructor with clinical experience would be helpful.

Suggested Resource Materials

CDT Book of Codes and Dental Procedures and Nomenclature: This provides students with numeric codes used to describe dentistry. The DENTRIX® Learning CD does not use actual CDT codes due to copyright issues. Students should be familiar with actual codes for charting.

TOPIC OUTLINE

1. Installing your DENTRIX® G4 Learning CD

   Registering your Software

   User's Guide

   Sample Practice

   Accessing DENTRIX®

   Web Sync and eSync Override

2. Patient Information

   Selecting a Patient

   Adding a New Patient

   Adding Medical Alerts

3. Patient Clinical Chart

4. Periodontal Charting

5. Appointment Book

   Find an Appointment Time

   Scheduling Appointments for an Existing Patient

   Scheduling Appointments for New Patients

   Rescheduling an Appointment

6. Adding Patient Photos

7. Tracking Patient Status

8. Prescriptions

TEACHING STRATEGIES

1. The key to success with the Learning CD is proper and complete installation. DENTRIX® has made the installation easy and this CD will run on Windows formats. Please encourage students to follow the steps carefully and to allow enough time. This is not a project for the end of a class period.

2. Students should understand that with the increase in "paperless" offices all dental team members must be knowledgeable regarding dental software.

3. Encourage students to work at their own pace. Some things will be easy, and others will be challenging—not unlike the rest of their dental studies. The skills do build on one another so spending the time to understand the process is important.

4. Students should relax and have fun: the Learning CD is very forgiving.

5. Your DENTRIX® Learning CD has a tutorial practice of 71 patients and an additional 29 can be added for a total of 100 patients. The best place to begin is to have students enter themselves, but it would be helpful to have some sample patient charts with information for students to enter as well.

6. Students should be encouraged to find answers within the User's Guide. Detailed instruction as to its location is found in the installation instructions. Working in an actual dental practice, they may need to be able to work independently.

Practice Management

SPECIFIC INSTRUCTIONAL OBJECTIVES

1. Demonstrate adding an employer to the DENTRIX® software.

2. Link a patient to the new employer.

3. Demonstrate adding an insurance company into the DENTRIX® software.

4. Link a patient to the new insurance company.

5. Write a patient letter using Quick Note.

6. Write a letter using the letter templates.

7. Post treatment to a patient's account.

8. Submit an insurance claim for completed patient treatment.

9. Submit a preauthorization.

10. Create a report showing patient referrals.

PREPARATORY

Personnel

The instructor providing guidance with the practice management portion of DENTRIX® should have a working knowledge of dental software, and an understanding of accounts receivable for a dental office, insurance, and correspondence.

TOPIC OUTLINE

1. Insurance

   Adding an Insurance Carrier

   Adding a Secondary Insurance Carrier

   Entering a New Insurance Carrier

2. Managing the Patient Ledger

   Adjusting an Account

   Editing or Deleting a Transaction

   Entering a Patient Payment

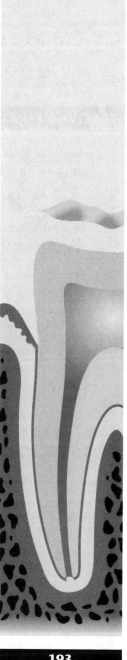

Entering an Insurance Payment

Walkout Statements

Quick Checkout

3. Correspondence

Writing Quick Letters

Recurring Care/Recall

Letters

Changing an Existing Letter

4. Organizing Information

Running Reports

Practice Goals Analysis

Using Practice Assistant

TEACHING STRATEGIES

1. Assist students in understanding how interconnected the elements of practice management software are and how mistakes compound themselves.

2. Encourage job shadowing where students could observe how computers are used in an office.

3. Have students update the charting they did in Part I–Patient Management as completed and follow the steps to send statements.

4. Have students practice writing business letters using DENTRIX®. Evaluate them for accuracy and appearance.

Evaluation of Chapter Knowledge Checklists

EVALUATION OF CHAPTER KNOWLEDGE CHECKLIST

1 Introduction to the Dental Profession

Knowledge	Good	Average	Poor
Recognizes the names of individuals who promoted education and organized dentistry.	○	○	○
Able to trace major discoveries and contributions to the history of dentistry.	○	○	○
Recognizes the major figures in dentistry today.	○	○	○
Defines and identifies DDS and DMD.	○	○	○
Able to identify the specialties in dentistry.	○	○	○
Able to describe the roles of the dental assistant, dental hygienist, and dental laboratory technician.	○	○	○
Knows each dental professional's educational requirements and professional organizations.	○	○	○

Grade: _____   Student's Initials _____   Instructor's Initials _____

EVALUATION OF CHAPTER KNOWLEDGE CHECKLIST

2 Psychology, Communication, and Multicultural Interaction

Knowledge	Good	Average	Poor
Defines psychology and paradigm.	○	○	○
Describes the components of the communication process.	○	○	○
Able to list the skills used in listening.	○	○	○
Able to differentiate the terms used for verbal and nonverbal communication.	○	○	○
Demonstrates and identifies the following body language used in nonverbal communication: spatial, posture, facial expression, gestures, and perception.	○	○	○
Understands how Maslow's hierarchy of needs is used and how it relates to communication in today's dental office.	○	○	○
Recognizes how defense mechanisms can inhibit communication.	○	○	○
Describes some general behaviors of multicultural patient populations.	○	○	○

Grade: _____   Student's Initials _____   Instructor's Initials _____

EVALUATION OF CHAPTER KNOWLEDGE CHECKLIST

3 Ethics, Jurisprudence, and the Health Information Portability and Accountability Act

Knowledge	Good	Average	Poor
Identifies the difference between civil and criminal law.	O	O	O
Able to define the Dental Practice Act and what it covers.	O	O	O
Able to identify who oversees the Dental Practice Act and how licenses for the dental field are obtained.	O	O	O
Able to define expanded functions.	O	O	O
Able to identify the components of a contract.	O	O	O
Identifies and defines fraud and due care, and provides examples of malpractice and torts.	O	O	O
Understands what fraud is.	O	O	O
Understands what can be done under the Good Samaritan Law.	O	O	O
Understands the responsibilities of the dental team in regard to dental records, implied and informed consent, subpoenas, and the statute of limitations.	O	O	O
Defines ethics and provides examples of the ADA and ADAA principles of ethics.	O	O	O
States how dentistry follows ethical principles in regard to advertising, professional fees and charges, and professional responsibilities and rights.	O	O	O
States how the HIPAA law has impacted the dental office and identifies the parameters of the law.	O	O	O
Able to identify how patient health information can be used and disclosed, and understands patient rights.	O	O	O
Understands the training required and how to be compliant with HIPAA laws.	O	O	O
Identifies CDT transactions and code sets.	O	O	O

Grade: _____   Student's Initials _____   Instructor's Initials _____

EVALUATION OF CHAPTER KNOWLEDGE CHECKLIST

4 Oral Health and Preventive Techniques

Knowledge	Good	Average	Poor
Discusses how plaque forms.	◯	◯	◯
Identifies the cause of plaque and its effects on the tooth.	◯	◯	◯
Discusses the importance of plaque control and describes oral hygiene aids.	◯	◯	◯
Demonstrates how to motivate patients to practice oral hygiene skills while instructing a variety of age groups.	◯	◯	◯
Differentiates between manual and automatic oral hygiene aids.	◯	◯	◯
Discusses how to use manual versus automatic oral hygiene aids appropriately.	◯	◯	◯
Performs the six toothbrushing techniques.	◯	◯	◯
Recognizes the various types of dental floss and aids.	◯	◯	◯
Performs the various techniques of flossing.	◯	◯	◯
Explains the role of fluoride in dentistry and how it is used.	◯	◯	◯
Understands the importance of fluoridation and its effect on tooth development during various development stages.	◯	◯	◯
Lists the various forms of fluoride and explains their applications.	◯	◯	◯
Properly prepares the patient for fluoride treatment.	◯	◯	◯

Grade: _____   Student's Initials _____   Instructor's Initials _____

EVALUATION OF CHAPTER KNOWLEDGE CHECKLIST

5 Nutrition

Knowledge	Good	Average	Poor
Explains the dental assistant's role when assisting patients with nutrition.	○	○	○
Lists the nutrients found in food that ensure meeting daily needs for essential nutrients.	○	○	○
Understands the important relationship of nutrients found in food and good nutrition in general for better oral health.	○	○	○
Explains the relationship between calories and basal metabolic rate.	○	○	○
Lists vitamins, minerals, and water, and describes how each functions in the body.	○	○	○
Able to discuss implications of eating disorders.	○	○	○
Explains how to interpret food labeling.	○	○	○

Grade: _____   Student's Initials _____   Instructor's Initials _____

EVALUATION OF CHAPTER KNOWLEDGE CHECKLIST

6 General Anatomy and Physiology

Knowledge	Good	Average	Poor
Identifies the body systems and understands body planes and their respective directions/orientations.	O	O	O
Identifies the cavities of the body.	O	O	O
Differentiates between body structure and cell formation.	O	O	O
Demonstrates an understanding of functions and divisions of the skeletal system.	O	O	O
Identifies bone composition and types of joints.	O	O	O
Identifies and describes the parts of the muscular system and respective functions.	O	O	O
Identifies and describes the structure of the nervous system and the functions of its components.	O	O	O
Identifies and describes the parts of the endocrine system and respective functions.	O	O	O
Understands dental concerns related to the reproductive system.	O	O	O
Identifies and describes the parts of the circulatory system and respective functions.	O	O	O
Demonstrates understanding of the parts of the digestive system and respective functions.	O	O	O
Identifies and describes the parts of the respiratory system and the functions of its components.	O	O	O
Identifies and describes the parts of the lymphatic and immune systems and respective functions.	O	O	O
Identifies and describes the parts of the integumentary system and respective functions.	O	O	O

Grade: _____   Student's Initials _____   Instructor's Initials _____

EVALUATION OF CHAPTER KNOWLEDGE CHECKLIST

7 Head and Neck Anatomy

Knowledge	Good	Average	Poor
Identifes and lists the anatomic landmarks of the face and oral cavity including the tongue, floor of the mouth, and salivary glands.	◯	◯	◯
Identifies the bones of the cranium and face.	◯	◯	◯
Recognizes maxilla and mandible landmarks.	◯	◯	◯
Identifies and lists the muscles of mastication, facial expression, floor of mouth, tongue, throat, neck, and shoulders, and describes their functions.	◯	◯	◯
Identifes and lists the nerves of the maxilla and the mandible.	◯	◯	◯
Identifes the arteries and veins of the head and neck.	◯	◯	◯

Grade: _____   Student's Initials _____   Instructor's Initials _____

EVALUATION OF CHAPTER KNOWLEDGE CHECKLIST

8 Embryology and Histology

Knowledge	Good	Average	Poor
Recognizes the three phases of pregnancy.	○	○	○
Lists the terms and times of phases of pregnancy.	○	○	○
Describes the developmental stages of the face during the zygote and embryo phases.	○	○	○
Defines and describes the stages in the tooth life cycle.	○	○	○
Describes the oral histology of the four primary tooth structures, and the location and function of each.	○	○	○
Identifies the microscopic structure and identifying marks of enamel, dentin, cementum, and pulp.	○	○	○
Lists the components of the periodontium related to tooth structure, support of hard and soft tissue, and the alveolar bone.	○	○	○
Lists the gingival fiber groups, gingiva, and alveolar mucosa and explains their relationship to the tooth.	○	○	○

Grade: _____   Student's Initials _____   Instructor's Initials _____

EVALUATION OF CHAPTER KNOWLEDGE CHECKLIST

9 Tooth Morphology

Knowledge	Good	Average	Poor
Differentiates between dental arches and quadrants and uses appropriate terminology.	○	○	○
Lists the deciduous teeth by name and location.	○	○	○
Knows the permanent dentition of teeth by name and location.	○	○	○
Describes the tooth eruption schedule for both primary and adult dentition.	○	○	○
Defines divisions of the tooth.	○	○	○
Differentiates between clinical and anatomical features of the tooth.	○	○	○
Identifies and describes the surface and location of each tooth.	○	○	○
Knows anatomical surfaces and identifies structures of each tooth.	○	○	○
Identifies individual teeth by anatomical landmarks and structures, including whether tooth is primary or adult.	○	○	○

Grade: _____   Student's Initials _____   Instructor's Initials _____

EVALUATION OF CHAPTER KNOWLEDGE CHECKLIST

10 Microbiology

Knowledge	Good	Average	Poor
Identifies key individuals in, and their contributions to, microbiology.	O	O	O
Differentiates between the two main groups of microorganisms that are identified in dentistry.	O	O	O
Describes staining procedures used to identify microorganisms.	O	O	O
Describes bacterial cell structure and discusses identification systems.	O	O	O
Differentiates among the characteristics of bacteria, protozoa, rickettsia, viruses, yeasts, and molds.	O	O	O
Lists the diseases of major concern to dental personnel.	O	O	O
Understands the importance of good health in preventing the transmission of infectious, and sometimes deadly, diseases.	O	O	O
Understands the importance of an alert dental assistant in recognizing potential exposure to contagious diseases and demonstrates proper safety precautions.	O	O	O
Describes the pathogen route and describes body defenses to prevent a disease.	O	O	O
Understands the functions of antibodies and a person's ability to resist pathogens or disease.	O	O	O
Lists the two normal routes of microorganism exposure in the dental office.	O	O	O

Grade: _____   Student's Initials _____   Instructor's Initials _____

EVALUATION OF CHAPTER KNOWLEDGE CHECKLIST

▐ **11 Infection Control**

Knowledge	Good	Average	Poor
Defines key vocabulary terms correctly.	○	○	○
Identifies and understands the importance of infection control in the dental setting.	○	○	○
Observes universal and standard precautions.	○	○	○
Demonstrates knowledge of OSHA-mandated training for all dental personnel.	○	○	○
Explains and describes the three primary routes in dentistry that transmit most microorganisms.	○	○	○
States and describes associated dental procedures that can expose the dental assistant to microbial transmission.	○	○	○
Identifies and demonstrates the components of personal protective equipment (PPE) and important safety precautions.	○	○	○
Applies knowledge in use of universal and standard precautions as they relate to cross-contamination, including dental records, handwashing, barriers, disinfectants, ultrasonic devices, sterilizers, and instrument storage.	○	○	○
Identifies and explains the use of disinfectants.	○	○	○
Identifies and knows how to operate the different types of sterilizers used in dentistry.	○	○	○
Performs proper bagging techniques and operation of sterilizers with various instruments.	○	○	○
Demonstrates proper use of sterilization monitors, including biological and process indicators.	○	○	○
Properly prepares the patient for use of preprocedure rinses.	○	○	○
Identifies and properly uses high-volume evacuation.	○	○	○
Properly explains the benefits of barriers and prepares the patient for the placement of rubber dams and other barrier items.	○	○	○

(continues)

EVALUATION OF CHAPTER KNOWLEDGE CHECKLIST

11 Infection Control *(continued)*

Knowledge	Good	Average	Poor
Explains and performs the correct protocol for infection control in all treatment areas both prior to seating the patient and at the end of treatment, and in the x-ray area and dental laboratory.	○	○	○
Recognizes the importance of quality infection control programs, instrument and operatory maintenance, and test controls.	○	○	○

Grade: _____   Student's Initials _____   Instructor's Initials _____

EVALUATION OF CHAPTER KNOWLEDGE CHECKLIST

12 Management of Hazardous Materials

Knowledge	Good	Average	Poor
Observes universal and standard precautions.	○	○	○
Defines key vocabulary terms correctly.	○	○	○
Can identify government regulatory agencies responsible for setting standards.	○	○	○
Able to explain the OSHA Bloodborne/Hazardous Material Standard and how to achieve compliance.	○	○	○
Able to explain the total compliance procedure in an occupational exposure incident.	○	○	○
Identifies body fluids and other potentially infectious materials (OPIMs).	○	○	○
Identifies and describes OSHA standards that ensure a safe work environment for dental employees, including physical equipment and mechanical devices used to safeguard employees.	○	○	○
Correctly and safely uses needle guards and disposes of needles.	○	○	○
Identifies and describes sharps containers.	○	○	○
Knows procedures for proper disposal of infectious waste.	○	○	○
Able to describe the hazardous communication standard and training requirements.	○	○	○
Differentiates between Hazardous Communication Standards and Bloodborne Standards.	○	○	○
Understands and explains the use of material safety data sheets and labeling methods.	○	○	○

Grade: _____   Student's Initials _____   Instructor's Initials _____

EVALUATION OF CHAPTER KNOWLEDGE CHECKLIST

13 Preparation for Patient Care

Knowledge	Good	Average	Poor
Understands the necessity for and function of the patient's medical history in dental treatment.	O	O	O
Defines the sections of a medical history.	O	O	O
Identifies and uses effective methods of interacting with patients.	O	O	O
Obtains a medical history from patient.	O	O	O
Understands issues of cultural sensitivity in taking a medical history.	O	O	O
Adapts communication to individual's ability to understand.	O	O	O
Documents accurately.	O	O	O
Explains different methods of charting/documentation.	O	O	O
Serves as a liaison between dentist and patient.	O	O	O
Defines and describes key terms relating to temperature, pulse, respiration, and blood pressure readings.	O	O	O
Knows anatomic locations of pulse sites and procedures to obtain pulse rate at each one.	O	O	O
Identifies normal and abnormal pulse rates.	O	O	O
Understands procedures for obtaining respiration rate.	O	O	O
Identifies normal and abnormal respiration rates.	O	O	O
Properly uses blood pressure equipment and understands measurement procedures.	O	O	O
Identifies normal and abnormal blood pressure readings, including factors that affect blood pressure.	O	O	O
Accurately records all measurements on the patient's chart.	O	O	O
Understands clinical evaluation and examination.	O	O	O

(continues)

EVALUATION OF CHAPTER KNOWLEDGE CHECKLIST

13 Preparation for Patient Care *(continued)*

Knowledge	Good	Average	Poor
Identifies the proper sequence of external examination during a clinical evaluation.	○	○	○
Identifies the proper sequence of internal examination during a clinical evaluation.	○	○	○

Grade: _____   Student's Initials _____   Instructor's Initials _____

EVALUATION OF CHAPTER KNOWLEDGE CHECKLIST

14 Dental Charting

Knowledge	Good	Average	Poor
Accurately describes the use of dental charting.	○	○	○
Differentiates among types of dental charts and various charting symbols for the oral cavity.	○	○	○
Able to chart both dentitions (adult and primary) using a variety of numbering systems.	○	○	○
Lists all cavity classifications and describes the anatomic structures involved.	○	○	○
Identifies common abbreviations used in cavity classifications.	○	○	○
Defines key terminology used during dental charting.	○	○	○
Performs proper use of color indicators and symbols represented in charting.	○	○	○

Grade: _____   Student's Initials _____   Instructor's Initials _____

EVALUATION OF CHAPTER KNOWLEDGE CHECKLIST

15 Pharmacology

Knowledge	Good	Average	Poor
Defines key vocabulary terms correctly.	◯	◯	◯
Describes the parts of a prescription, including Latin abbreviations.	◯	◯	◯
Understands what the federal Comprehensive Drug Abuse Prevention and Control Act of 1970 entails.	◯	◯	◯
Can define the law in terms of administering, prescribing, and dispensing drugs.	◯	◯	◯
Differentiates between brand-name and generic drugs.	◯	◯	◯
Can explain the use of the *Physician's Desk Reference* (PDR) and can locate a drug and its chemical description.	◯	◯	◯
Lists and explains the route a drug takes when administered.	◯	◯	◯
Able to list commonly abused drugs and recognize their effects.	◯	◯	◯
Lists and explains the differences among amphetamines, hallucinogens, and barbiturates.	◯	◯	◯
Able to identify and explain medications that a patient may receive to alleviate anxiety and discomfort from dental treatment.	◯	◯	◯
Accurately documents all medications given to the patient.	◯	◯	◯

Grade: _____   Student's Initials _____   Instructor's Initials _____

EVALUATION OF CHAPTER KNOWLEDGE CHECKLIST

16 Emergency Management

Knowledge	Good	Average	Poor
Recognizes emergency situations.	◯	◯	◯
Understands the need for emergency preparedness and the function of emergency medical service.	◯	◯	◯
Able to perform CPR in emergencies.	◯	◯	◯
Understands legal and health considerations of emergency care.	◯	◯	◯
Understands the necessity of providing emergency care only within the scope of training and knowledge.	◯	◯	◯
Can assemble an emergency kit and crash cart.	◯	◯	◯
Understands the use of standard precautions in emergency situations.	◯	◯	◯
Identifies sudden illnesses such as syncope, seizures, diabetes mellitus, and anaphylactic and allergic reactions.	◯	◯	◯
Recognizes heart attack and priorities for immediate emergency care.	◯	◯	◯
Recognizes a cerebral vascular accident (stroke) and priorities for immediate emergency care.	◯	◯	◯
Can identify and name steps for performing these emergency procedures: Airway obstruction Avulsed tooth Heimlich maneuver Rescue breathing Infant, teenage, and adult CPR	◯ ◯ ◯ ◯ ◯	◯ ◯ ◯ ◯ ◯	◯ ◯ ◯ ◯ ◯
Has a basic understanding of the use of a pulse oximeter.	◯	◯	◯
Has a basic understanding for the use of capnography.	◯	◯	◯
Has a basic understanding for the use of electrocardiography.	◯	◯	◯

Grade: _____   Student's Initials _____   Instructor's Initials _____

EVALUATION OF CHAPTER KNOWLEDGE CHECKLIST

17 Introduction to the Dental Office and Basic Chairside Assisting

Knowledge	Good	Average	Poor
Exhibits empathy with patient experience in the dental setting.	○	○	○
Ability to identify members of the dental health team.	○	○	○
Understands the concepts of the dental assistant's role.	○	○	○
Identifies tasks associated with opening and closing the facility.	○	○	○
Recognizes the importance of the reception and business office staff and areas.	○	○	○
Relates the physical environment of the facility to patient care and comfort.	○	○	○
Relates the physical environment of the facility to optimal function and efficiency.	○	○	○
Understands the purpose of the ADA, and can describe methods of compliance.	○	○	○
Understands the importance of teamwork.	○	○	○
Understands the steps to seat a patient for treatment.	○	○	○
Identifies the instruments and supplies required to prepare a patient for treatment.	○	○	○
Properly places patient in operating position.	○	○	○
Recalls the method of examination, including instruments, and the operator and assistant positions.	○	○	○
Respects the patient and attends to the patient's special needs during care.	○	○	○
Prepares and maintains examination and treatment areas.	○	○	○
Understands steps for dismissing the patient after treatment.	○	○	○

Grade: _____   Student's Initials _____   Instructor's Initials _____

EVALUATION OF CHAPTER KNOWLEDGE CHECKLIST

18 Basic Chairside Instruments and Tray Systems

Knowledge	Good	Average	Poor
Defines the parts of an instrument.	O	O	O
States and describes how an instrument is identified.	O	O	O
Defines the parts of a bur.	O	O	O
Explains the different categories of dental burs.	O	O	O
Understands the necessary functions of different burs.	O	O	O
States and describes the use and adaptation of fiber-optic light sources and high-speed and low-speed handpieces.	O	O	O
Demonstrates competent handpiece identification and knowledge of various attachments.	O	O	O
Identifies the sequence of instrumentation, supplies, and equipment needed during use of abrasives.	O	O	O
Observes all standard precautions and applies principles of aseptic technique.	O	O	O

Grade: _____   Student's Initials _____   Instructor's Initials _____

EVALUATION OF CHAPTER KNOWLEDGE CHECKLIST

19 Instrument Transfer and Maintaining the Operating Field

Knowledge	Good	Average	Poor
Demonstrates the ability to perform grasps and positions during instrument transfers.	○	○	○
Demonstrates the ability to maintain a clear operating field through HVE use.	○	○	○
Observes all standard precautions and applies the principles of aseptic technique.	○	○	○
Respects the patient and attends to the patient's needs during care.	○	○	○

Grade: _____   Student's Initials _____   Instructor's Initials _____

EVALUATION OF CHAPTER KNOWLEDGE CHECKLIST

20 Anesthesia and Sedation

Knowledge	Good	Average	Poor
Understands the considerations of anesthetic selection to control pain and for the anxious patient.	○	○	○
Understands the ratios and proportions of topical and local anesthetics.	○	○	○
Lists guidelines to follow when preparing anesthetics.	○	○	○
Describes the procedures for the safe disposal of syringes, needles, and biohazard materials.	○	○	○
Describes site selection for the administration of injections.	○	○	○
Understands allergic reactions.	○	○	○
Describes nitrous oxide sedation medication and proper administration.	○	○	○
Exhibits communication skills in administering medications to patients.	○	○	○
Accurately documents the medications given to patients.	○	○	○
Complies with federal and state regulations in the administration and disposal of controlled substances.	○	○	○
Identifies the equipment and supplies used to prepare the patient for topical, local, and nitrous oxide anesthetics.	○	○	○
Describes supplemental techniques and site locations for anesthesia administration.	○	○	○

Grade: _____   Student's Initials _____   Instructor's Initials _____

EVALUATION OF CHAPTER KNOWLEDGE CHECKLIST

21 Introduction to Dental Radiography and Equipment

Knowledge	Good	Average	Poor
Demonstrates the ability to trace the discovery of x-rays and radiological contributions to the history of dentistry.	◯	◯	◯
Identifies the properties of radiation and the biological effects of radiation exposure.	◯	◯	◯
Understands the crucial role of safety precautions and quality control when using radiation.	◯	◯	◯
Identifies the parts of the dental x-ray unit and describes their functions.	◯	◯	◯
Describes how an x-ray is produced.	◯	◯	◯
Describes the composition of dental x-ray film.	◯	◯	◯
Identifies the sizes and types of dental x-ray films.	◯	◯	◯
Understands the concerns of dental x-ray film storage.	◯	◯	◯
Understands that the patient record includes storage of x-rays and associated legal implications.	◯	◯	◯
Documents all radiographic exposures according to state statutes of limitations.	◯	◯	◯
Identifies quality assurance policies and standard procedures that dental offices follow to ensure quality radiographs.	◯	◯	◯

Grade: _____   Student's Initials _____   Instructor's Initials _____

EVALUATION OF CHAPTER KNOWLEDGE CHECKLIST

22 Production and Evaluation of Dental Radiographs

Knowledge	Good	Average	Poor
Differentiates between intraoral and extraoral x-ray exposures and production exposures.	O	O	O
Demonstrates the ability to differentiate and explain the production of paralleling and bisecting exposures.	O	O	O
Understands ways to produce quality radiographic exposures on a variety of patients.	O	O	O
Understands the factors affecting accurate radiographic exposures.	O	O	O
Identifies and lists common production errors.	O	O	O
Explains the processing techniques of, and differentiates between, manual and automatic processors.	O	O	O
Knows the general safety rules of processing methods.	O	O	O
Identifies processing solutions and their compositions.	O	O	O
Understands that the patient record includes storage of x-rays and associated legal implications.	O	O	O

Grade: _____   Student's Initials _____   Instructor's Initials _____

EVALUATION OF CHAPTER KNOWLEDGE CHECKLIST

23 Extraoral and Digital Radiography

Knowledge	Good	Average	Poor
Differentiates between intraoral and extraoral x-ray exposures and production exposures.	○	○	○
Identifies and describes extraoral film.	○	○	○
Accurately exposes extraoral film.	○	○	○
Differentiates between normal and abnormal radiographic landmarks.	○	○	○
Identifies quality assurance policies and standard procedures that dental offices follow to ensure quality radiographs.	○	○	○
Recognizes the role of digital imaging systems in dentistry.	○	○	○
Accurately exposes x-rays using digital radiography.	○	○	○
Defines key radiograph interpretation terminology relating to the tooth and the surrounding tissues.	○	○	○
Identifies key landmarks of the maxilla and the mandible.	○	○	○
Recognizes conditions or artifacts that may appear on x-rays.	○	○	○
Understands the uses and benefits of 3-D imaging.	○	○	○
Can describe the function and use of hand-held imaging devices.	○	○	○

Grade: _____   Student's Initials _____   Instructor's Initials _____

EVALUATION OF CHAPTER KNOWLEDGE CHECKLIST

24 Endodontics

Knowledge	Good	Average	Poor
Correctly defines key vocabulary terms associated with endodontics.	○	○	○
Differentiates between pulpal and periapical disease.	○	○	○
Lists the general steps in endodontic diagnosis.	○	○	○
Recognizes endodontic instruments and identifies their functions in the dental procedure.	○	○	○
Recognizes endodontic materials and identifies their functions in the dental procedure.	○	○	○
Lists the nine general steps in root canal therapy.	○	○	○
Explains and/or demonstrates the role of the dental assistant during the root canal procedure.	○	○	○
Explains the process of retreatment for an endodontically treated tooth.	○	○	○
Differentiates between apicoectomy, root amputation, and hemisection.	○	○	○
Recognizes the instruments used during the three surgical endodontic procedures and explains their functions in each procedure.	○	○	○

Grade: _____   Student's Initials _____   Instructor's Initials _____

EVALUATION OF CHAPTER KNOWLEDGE CHECKLIST

25 Oral and Maxillofacial Surgery

Knowledge	Good	Average	Poor
Correctly defines key vocabulary terms.	○	○	○
Understands the branch of dentistry that focuses on the diagnosis and treatment of diseases, injuries, and malformations.	○	○	○
Recognizes various surgical instruments and describes their functions.	○	○	○
Observes all standard precautions and applies principles of aseptic techniques.	○	○	○
Understands the standard precautions of applied aseptic techniques as they relate to a sterile surgical work environment.	○	○	○
Defines the terms of informed consent.	○	○	○
States the procedures involved in patient evaluation before oral surgery.	○	○	○
Lists the five steps in preparing a patient for surgical treatment.	○	○	○
Recognizes the instruments involved in routine or uncomplicated extractions, multiple extractions, alveoplasty, impacted teeth, and biopsy procedures.	○	○	○
States instrument functions in each procedure and dental assistant responsibilities for each.	○	○	○
Explains the postoperative home-care instructions given to patients, including what to expect, what to do, and things to avoid.	○	○	○
Differentiates between subperiosteal and endosteal dental implants, explaining their purposes and uses in dental treatment.	○	○	○
Understands the hospital protocol for an oral maxillofacial surgeon and recognizes the types of patients who might require hospitalization for dental treatment.	○	○	○

(continues)

EVALUATION OF CHAPTER KNOWLEDGE CHECKLIST

25 Oral and Maxillofacial Surgery *(continued)*

Suture Removal	Good	Average	Poor
Explains the function of sutures and where they are placed.	○	○	○
Lists the equipment and supplies needed for suture removal.	○	○	○
Explains suture site, assessment of tissue condition, and healing process.	○	○	○
Describes assessment criteria for postoperative patient care.	○	○	○
Understands, recognizes, and differentiates basic patterns of suturing.	○	○	○
Explains identification of suture patterns and determines appropriate removal procedure.	○	○	○
Explains the 10-step guide to suture removal.	○	○	○

Grade: _____   Student's Initials _____   Instructor's Initials _____

EVALUATION OF CHAPTER KNOWLEDGE CHECKLIST

26 Oral Pathology

Knowledge	Good	Average	Poor
Correctly defines key vocabulary terms.	○	○	○
Understands oral diseases, their origins, and their effects on the body.	○	○	○
Explains and/or demonstrates the role and reporting responsibilities of the dental assistant during patient observation.	○	○	○
Describes the distinctive process of inflammation.	○	○	○
Identifies oral lesions according to their distinctive traits and particular regions or surface areas.	○	○	○
Describes oral diseases caused by microorganisms and how they are revealed through the lesion.	○	○	○
Identifies the physical agents that can cause oral clinical manifestations and differentiates them from trauma-induced lesions.	○	○	○
Describes the oral diseases related to lesions caused by chemical agents common in dentistry.	○	○	○
Lists and explains three oral conditions caused by hormonal disturbances.	○	○	○
Differentiates the oral conditions related to developmental disturbances from anomalies caused by outside agents.	○	○	○
Explains the effect of poor or improper diet on the condition of the oral cavity.	○	○	○
Explains and/or demonstrates the role of the dental assistant during the clinical examination for any premalignant lesion.	○	○	○
Lists the early warning signs of oral cancer.	○	○	○
Differentiates the characteristics of at least seven lesions that have significant potential for becoming malignant.	○	○	○

(continues)

EVALUATION OF CHAPTER KNOWLEDGE CHECKLIST

26 Oral Pathology *(continued)*

Knowledge	Good	Average	Poor
Possesses working knowledge of the conditions, manifestations, opportunistic infections, and malignancies that may appear in AIDS patients.	○	○	○
Understands that healthy people can combat most microorganisms, but that those who suffer from suppressed immune systems cannot.	○	○	○
Explains six known miscellaneous disorders affecting the oral cavity.	○	○	○

Grade: _____   Student's Initials _____   Instructor's Initials _____

EVALUATION OF CHAPTER KNOWLEDGE CHECKLIST

27 Orthodontics

Knowledge	Good	Average	Poor
Identifies auxiliary members of the orthodontic team.	◯	◯	◯
Recognizes the importance of the receptionist and business office staff and areas.	◯	◯	◯
Relates the physical environment of the facility to the specialty of orthodontics and orthodontic patient care and comfort.	◯	◯	◯
Relates the physical environment of the facility to optimal function and efficiency.	◯	◯	◯
Correctly defines key vocabulary terms.	◯	◯	◯
Differentiates between occlusion and malocclusion.	◯	◯	◯
Explains the Edward Angle system of classifying malocclusion.	◯	◯	◯
Explains the etiology (causes) of malocclusion.	◯	◯	◯
Understands and describes preventive, interceptive, and corrective orthodontia.	◯	◯	◯
Lists the principles of tooth movement.	◯	◯	◯
Lists the steps in preorthodontic treatment, including diagnostic records and processing appointments.	◯	◯	◯
Describes the consultation appointment and roles of the orthodontist and patient.	◯	◯	◯
Differentiates between the preorthodontic treatment appointment and the consultation appointment.	◯	◯	◯
Recognizes the variety of fixed orthodontic appliances.	◯	◯	◯
Differentiates between special and routine fixed orthodontic appliances and states their purposes and uses.	◯	◯	◯

(continues)

EVALUATION OF CHAPTER KNOWLEDGE CHECKLIST

27 Orthodontics *(continued)*

Knowledge	Good	Average	Poor
Recognizes the variety of removable orthodontic appliances and states their purposes and uses.	○	○	○
Identifies and provides the functions of the instruments used during the placement and removal of elastic and steel separators, brass wire procedures, direct bonding of brackets, placement of arch wire and ligament ties, and completion appointment procedures.	○	○	○
Explains and/or demonstrates the role of the dental assistant during basic orthodontic procedures.	○	○	○
Identifies and states the functions of materials needed in orthodontic procedures.	○	○	○
Describes the stages of orthodontic treatment.	○	○	○
Describes the steps in a completion appointment procedure.	○	○	○
Explains the procedures for removing orthodontic appliances and how teeth are retained in position.	○	○	○

Grade: _____   Student's Initials _____   Instructor's Initials _____

EVALUATION OF CHAPTER KNOWLEDGE CHECKLIST

28 Pediatric Dentistry and Enamel Sealants

Knowledge	Good	Average	Poor
Understands pediatric dentistry as a specialty.	○	○	○
Identifies members of the pediatric dental team and the special considerations of working with children.	○	○	○
Relates the physical environment of the facility to the "open bay" concept and inclusion of a "quiet room."	○	○	○
Correctly defines key vocabulary terms.	○	○	○
Understands the behavior of children at various ages, and can identify ways to establish relationships with children.	○	○	○
Explains the "tell, show, and do" technique and other behavior management methods.	○	○	○
Identifies methods for helping parents or guardians prepare children for dental care.	○	○	○
Lists the common procedures in pediatric dentistry.	○	○	○
Recognizes the instrumentation for pediatric procedures and describes its function.	○	○	○
Recognizes the equipment unique to pediatric dentistry.	○	○	○
Explains the emergency treatment of fractured teeth, traumatic intrusion, displaced teeth, and avulsed teeth.	○	○	○
Lists the types of child abuse and associated injuries that might be identified in the dental office.	○	○	○
Understands the laws regarding child abuse and the procedures for reporting a suspected abuse case.	○	○	○

(continues)

EVALUATION OF CHAPTER KNOWLEDGE CHECKLIST

28 Pediatric Dentistry and Enamel Sealants *(continued)*

Enamel Sealants	Good	Average	Poor
Understands the purpose of enamel sealants and where they are placed.	○	○	○
Lists the indications and contraindications of placing sealants.	○	○	○
Explains the dental assistant's role in placing sealants.	○	○	○
Differentiates between chemically cured and light-cured sealant materials.	○	○	○
Explains and defines the procedures of sealant placement.	○	○	○

Grade: _____   Student's Initials _____   Instructor's Initials _____

EVALUATION OF CHAPTER KNOWLEDGE CHECKLIST

29 Periodontics and Coronal Polish

Knowledge	Good	Average	Poor
Understands the dental specialty practice that deals with the symptoms, probable causes, diagnosis, and treatment of periodontal disease.	○	○	○
Identifies members of the periodontal dental team and explains their roles.	○	○	○
Lists and describes steps in the periodontal diagnosis procedure during a patient's first visit.	○	○	○
Explains etiology of periodontal disease and involvement of the structures of the periodontium.	○	○	○
Differentiates between gingivitis and periodontitis, and explains the course and characteristics of each disease.	○	○	○
Correctly defines key vocabulary terms.	○	○	○
Recognizes periodontal instruments and their functions in each procedure.	○	○	○
Recognizes nonsurgical periodontal procedures and identifies the instrumentation and related functions of each procedure.	○	○	○
Explains the role of the dental assistant during surgical periodontal procedures.	○	○	○
Differentiates among gingivectomy, gingivoplasty, and periodontal flap surgery.	○	○	○
Differentiates among osseous surgery, mucogingival surgery, gingival grafting, and frenectomy.	○	○	○
Lists and describes the types of periodontal dressings.	○	○	○
Explains and/or demonstrates how periodontal dressings are prepared, placed, and removed.	○	○	○
Explains the procedure for maintaining the status of periodontal health after surgery and the patient's role in home oral hygiene routines.	○	○	○

(continues)

EVALUATION OF CHAPTER KNOWLEDGE CHECKLIST

29 Periodontics and Coronal Polish *(continued)*

Coronal Polishing	Good	Average	Poor
Explains rationales for performing coronal polishing.	○	○	○
Describes indications and contraindications for coronal polishing.	○	○	○
Describes methods for recognizing and differentiating various dental deposits and stains.	○	○	○
Identifies various types of abrasives and describes their individual characteristics that determine abrasiveness.	○	○	○
Describes and explains the equipment and materials used to perform coronal polishing.	○	○	○
Describes how to maintain the oral cavity during coronal polishing.	○	○	○
Identifies various polishing aids and describes their function.	○	○	○
Explains the steps in the coronal polishing procedure.	○	○	○

Grade: _____   Student's Initials _____   Instructor's Initials _____

EVALUATION OF CHAPTER KNOWLEDGE CHECKLIST

30 Fixed Prosthodontics and Gingival Retraction

Knowledge	Good	Average	Poor
Understands the dental specialty that deals with the replacement of missing teeth or parts of teeth with extensive restorations.	○	○	○
Lists and describes the types of fixed prostheses and their functions.	○	○	○
Lists and describes evaluations the dentist performs on patients to determine if they are candidates for fixed prostheses.	○	○	○
Differentiates among dental materials used in porcelain veneers, temporaries, and final cementation stages, and states their functions and purposes during specific procedures.	○	○	○
Explains the role of the laboratory technician during the fabrication of fixed prostheses.	○	○	○
Correctly defines key vocabulary terms.	○	○	○
Explains the role of the dental assistant during all phases of fixed prosthodontic treatment.	○	○	○
Differentiates among retention techniques for core buildup, retention pin, and post-retained cores.	○	○	○
Explains the osseointegration process and use of the implant-retained prostheses.	○	○	○
Describes home-care instructions for properly maintained fixed prostheses.	○	○	○

(continues)

EVALUATION OF CHAPTER KNOWLEDGE CHECKLIST

30 Fixed Prosthodontics and Gingival Retraction *(continued)*

Gingival Retraction	Good	Average	Poor
Explains the function of gingival retraction.	○	○	○
Describe the types of gingival retraction techniques including: mechanical, chemical, and surgical methods.	○	○	○
Explain retraction systems that are used as alternatives to placing retraction cord.	○	○	○
Describes procedural steps to place and remove gingival retraction cord.	○	○	○

Grade: _____ Student's Initials _____ Instructor's Initials _____

EVALUATION OF CHAPTER KNOWLEDGE CHECKLIST

31 Cosmetic Dentistry and Teeth Whitening

Knowledge	Good	Average	Poor
Describes cosmetic dentistry and compares it to general dentistry.	○	○	○
Explains who performs cosmetic dentistry and education requirements.	○	○	○
Describes the dental assistant's role when working in a cosmetic dental practice.	○	○	○
Explains the scope of cosmetic dentistry and the fundamental principles involved in creating the perfect smile.	○	○	○
Describes the basic elements of psychology and sociology that are considered for cosmetic treatment.	○	○	○
Explains what the patient should consider when selecting a dentist for cosmetic treatment.	○	○	○
Describes specific procedures performed in cosmetic dentistry, including diagnosis and treatment planning, and completing legal forms and documentation.	○	○	○
Explains the role of oral photography in cosmetic dentistry.	○	○	○
Identifes oral photography equipment.	○	○	○
Describes how the patient is positioned for taking photographs that are needed in cosmetic dental treatment.	○	○	○

(continues)

EVALUATION OF CHAPTER KNOWLEDGE CHECKLIST

31 Cosmetic Dentistry and Teeth Whitening *(continued)*

Knowledge	Good	Average	Poor
Describes the why and how of soft tissue surgery in cosmetic dentistry and how lasers and electrosurgery are involved.	○	○	○
Explains why the dental team needs to know about occlusion and cosmetic dentistry.	○	○	○
List the types of restorations and materials used in cosmetic restorations.	○	○	○
Describes marketing techniques for cosmetic dentistry.	○	○	○
Understands and describes the aesthetic benefits of safe and effective whitening methods.	○	○	○
Differentiates among dental office, at-home, and walking whitening techniques.	○	○	○
Explains the procedural steps to accomplish each of the above three techniques.	○	○	○
Explains the information provided to patients on steps, outcomes, patient responsibilities, and precautions related to whitening.	○	○	○

Grade: _____   Student's Initials _____   Instructor's Initials _____

EVALUATION OF CHAPTER KNOWLEDGE CHECKLIST

32 Removable Prosthodontics

Knowledge	Good	Average	Poor
Correctly defines key vocabulary terms.	○	○	○
Lists and describes the goals of removable prostheses.	○	○	○
Explains required patient considerations for successful treatment using removable prostheses.	○	○	○
Describes and/or demonstrates the main functions of the dental assistant in removable prosthetic procedures.	○	○	○
Describes the steps in the diagnostic appointment and explains the materials needed.	○	○	○
Explains the steps of the consultation appointment and names five setup items prepared for the dentist.	○	○	○
Explains the advantages and disadvantages of the partial denture.	○	○	○
Identifies and explains the components of the partial denture.	○	○	○
Explains the six-step appointment procedure for a partial denture and the content of each step.	○	○	○
Defines complete denture.	○	○	○
Explains the evaluation process of a patient being considered for a complete denture.	○	○	○
Identifies and describes the components of a complete denture.	○	○	○
Explains the eight-step appointment procedure for a complete denture.	○	○	○
Describes the types and required steps of denture reline procedures.	○	○	○
Explains the steps and materials needed for a denture repair.	○	○	○
Lists and describes the care and considerations of polishing removable prostheses.	○	○	○
Explains advantages and disadvantages of the overdenture.	○	○	○

Grade: _____   Student's Initials _____   Instructor's Initials _____

EVALUATION OF CHAPTER KNOWLEDGE CHECKLIST

33 Dental Cements, Bases, Liners, and Bonding Agents

Knowledge	Good	Average	Poor
Describes the common types of dental restorative materials and how they are divided and categorized according to their function.	◯	◯	◯
Identifies regulating agencies overseeing dental materials.	◯	◯	◯
Describes the role of each regulating agency and its responsibilities with respect to function, safety, and use.	◯	◯	◯
Describes the dental assistant's role when working with dental restorative materials.	◯	◯	◯
Describes properties of dental materials.	◯	◯	◯
Differentiates between the two sections of dental materials used to restore teeth.	◯	◯	◯
Recognizes and differentiates between the types of dental cements.	◯	◯	◯
Describes the eight dental cements by properties, composition, use, and manipulation.	◯	◯	◯
Differentiates between dentin and enamel bonding.	◯	◯	◯
Explains bonding application and manipulation.	◯	◯	◯
Lists and explains cavity preparation terminology.	◯	◯	◯
Lists the steps and explains the considerations for cavity preparation.	◯	◯	◯

(continues)

EVALUATION OF CHAPTER KNOWLEDGE CHECKLIST

33 Dental Cements, Bases, Liners, and Bonding Agents *(continued)*

Placing Bases, Liners, and Varnishes	Good	Average	Poor
Differentiates cavity preparations to assess their relationship for pulp protection.	○	○	○
Describes various options of pulp protection material, and differentiates between categories and their treatment applications.	○	○	○
Explains the assessment process in selecting cavity liners in terms of their purpose and placement procedures.	○	○	○
Differentiates between cavity varnish and cavity liners.	○	○	○
Explains the purpose and placement procedure for cavity varnish.	○	○	○
Explains the purpose and placement procedure of various cement bases.	○	○	○

Grade: _____   Student's Initials _____   Instructor's Initials _____

EVALUATION OF CHAPTER KNOWLEDGE CHECKLIST

34 Restorative Materials, Dental Dam, Matrix, and Wedge

Knowledge	Good	Average	Poor
Describes the common types of dental restorative materials, and how they are categorized according to their function.	◯	◯	◯
Describes the dental assistant's role when working with dental restorative materials.	◯	◯	◯
Differentiates between the two sections of dental materials used to restore teeth.	◯	◯	◯
Recognizes and differentiates between amalgam and composites.	◯	◯	◯
Explains the application of amalgam and composites.	◯	◯	◯
Lists and recognizes the armamentarium for an amalgam restoration.	◯	◯	◯
Lists and describes the steps for an amalgam restoration.	◯	◯	◯
Lists and recognizes the armamentarium for a composite restoration.	◯	◯	◯
Lists and describes the steps for a composite restoration.	◯	◯	◯
Describes and explains the use of glass ionomer, resin, resin-reinforced glass ionomer, and compomer restorative materials.	◯	◯	◯
Understands and explains the reasons that a dental dam is used and the responsibilities of those who perform this function.	◯	◯	◯
Explains the advantages and disadvantages of the dental dam.	◯	◯	◯
Recognizes the armamentarium prescribed for a dental dam procedure and can explain the functions of each element.	◯	◯	◯
Describes patient preparation for dental dam placement, explains the evaluation of the selected isolation area, and performs the setup procedure for dental dam placement.	◯	◯	◯

(continues)

EVALUATION OF CHAPTER KNOWLEDGE CHECKLIST

34 Restorative Materials, Dental Dam, Matrix, and Wedge (continued)

Knowledge	Good	Average	Poor
Lists and performs the steps in placing the dental dam, while demonstrating proper precautions.	○	○	○
Lists and performs the steps in removing the dental dam, while demonstrating proper precautions.	○	○	○
Lists and performs the steps in the dental dam procedure for a child patient, while demonstrating proper precautions.	○	○	○
Explains and describes the uses and types of matrices.	○	○	○
Identifies the parts, functions, effective placement, and removal of the Tofflemire matrix.	○	○	○
Performs and describes placement and removal of the strip matrix.	○	○	○
Identifies the parts, and performs and describes placement and removal of the automatrix.	○	○	○
Identifies the parts, and performs and describes placement and removal of sectional matrix systems.	○	○	○

Grade: _____   Student's Initials _____   Instructor's Initials _____

EVALUATION OF CHAPTER KNOWLEDGE CHECKLIST

35 Laboratory Materials and Techniques

Knowledge	Good	Average	Poor
Recognizes materials used in the dental laboratory and accurately performs related procedures.	○	○	○
Applies knowledge accurately while preparing, taking, and removing alginate impressions.	○	○	○
Defines key terms related to laboratory materials and techniques.	○	○	○
Accurately applies knowledge and skills in preparing irreversible hydrocolloid impression material.	○	○	○
Accurately applies knowledge and skills in preparing various elastomeric impression materials (polysulfide, silicone, and polyether), and explains their respective applications.	○	○	○
Accurately applies knowledge and skills in using gypsum products (Types I to V).	○	○	○
Accurately performs and explains pouring and trimming a patient's alginate impression (diagnostic cast).	○	○	○
Demonstrates and explains the use of a dental articulator for dental casts or study models.	○	○	○
Recognizes and differentiates among types of dental waxes and explains the uses of each.	○	○	○
Accurately applies knowledge and skills in fabricating custom trays (acrylic resin self-curing, light-curing, vacuum-formed, and thermoplastic).	○	○	○
Accurately applies knowledge and skills to contour prefabricated temporary crowns and to fabricate and fit custom temporary restorations.	○	○	○

Grade: _____   Student's Initials _____   Instructor's Initials _____

EVALUATION OF CHAPTER KNOWLEDGE CHECKLIST

36 Dental Office Management

Knowledge	Good	Average	Poor
Describes the roles of the dental receptionist and business office staff and their related responsibilities.	O	O	O
Understands effective strategies for marketing as a means to attract and retain patients.	O	O	O
Understands the principles of successful telephone communications.	O	O	O
Describes the proper procedures for answering an incoming call.	O	O	O
Understands telephone procedures for new and existing patient appointments.	O	O	O
Demonstrates ability to take and record telephone messages.	O	O	O
Understands the use of communication technology such as fax machines, answering systems, e-mail, and copying.	O	O	O
Able to receive, prioritize, organize, and transmit information.	O	O	O
Demonstrates ability to make outgoing calls.	O	O	O
Identifies types of computer hardware.	O	O	O
Defines key vocabulary terms.	O	O	O
Distinguishes between software and hardware.	O	O	O
Identifies categories of applications software and can describe the purpose of each.	O	O	O
Understands how computers enhance office efficiency and gives examples of specific methods.	O	O	O
Applies database management concepts to a dental setting.	O	O	O
Can relate relevant ergonomic theories and give guidelines for setting up ergonomic workstations.	O	O	O

(continues)

EVALUATION OF CHAPTER KNOWLEDGE CHECKLIST

36 Dental Office Management *(continued)*

Knowledge	Good	Average	Poor
Can discuss the increasing role of computers in dentistry for both clinical and administrative tasks.	○	○	○
Able to establish an appointment matrix.	○	○	○
Prepares daily appointment sheet.	○	○	○
Prepares daily worksheet.	○	○	○
Understands importance of scheduling patient appointments.	○	○	○
Understands basic considerations in scheduling appointments.	○	○	○
Recognizes the importance of communications skills in the scheduling process.	○	○	○
Recalls common equipment and supplies used for dental records management.	○	○	○
Names and describes basic rules for filing.	○	○	○
States the reasons for accurately maintaining dental office files.	○	○	○
Understands color-coding filing systems.	○	○	○
Understands rules of confidentiality when handling patient's dental records.	○	○	○
Demonstrates ability to manage accounts receivable.	○	○	○
Demonstrates ability to manage accounts payable.	○	○	○
Accurately completes a charge slip.	○	○	○
Able to use manual bookkeeping pegboard system.	○	○	○
Able to establish, track, and balance a day sheet.	○	○	○

(continues)

EVALUATION OF CHAPTER KNOWLEDGE CHECKLIST

36 Dental Office Management *(continued)*

Knowledge	Good	Average	Poor
Displays ability to write and record checks, and reconcile accounts.	○	○	○
Documents various financial forms correctly.	○	○	○
Correctly spells difficult and commonly misspelled and misused words.	○	○	○
Understands and can define basic accounting terms.	○	○	○
Recognizes the challenges of converting from a manual to a computerized accounting system.	○	○	○

Grade: _____   Student's Initials _____   Instructor's Initials _____

EVALUATION OF CHAPTER KNOWLEDGE CHECKLIST

37 Employment Strategies

Knowledge	Good	Average	Poor
Can explain the four pathways to obtaining DANB certification.	○	○	○
Identifies the benefits of certification.	○	○	○
Correctly defines key vocabulary terms.	○	○	○
Understands the qualifications required to sit for the DANB certification exam.	○	○	○
Describes personal short-range and long-range goals.	○	○	○
Describes the role of goal setting.	○	○	○
Lists sources for locating open employment positions.	○	○	○
Explains the purpose and content of a cover letter.	○	○	○
Identifies the standard format used to develop a cover letter.	○	○	○
Explains the purpose and content of a résumé.	○	○	○
Explains the interview process.	○	○	○
Demonstrates effective interview behavior.	○	○	○
Can receive, prioritize, organize, and transmit information during an interview.	○	○	○
Understands the importance of displaying professionalism.	○	○	○
Identifies benefits of a follow-up letter.	○	○	○
Uses self-assessment techniques to determine optimal employment goals.	○	○	○
Recalls correct method to terminate employment.	○	○	○

Grade: _____   Student's Initials _____   Instructor's Initials _____

EVALUATION OF CHAPTER KNOWLEDGE CHECKLIST

Patient Management

Knowledge	Successful	Needs Assistance
Accesses DENTRIX®.	○	○
Demonstrates multiple ways to select a patient.	○	○
Ability to add a new patient.	○	○
Adds employer to patient information.	○	○
Ability to add additional family members.	○	○
Explains or shows how to add a photo.	○	○
Charts new treatment.	○	○
Charts existing treatment.	○	○
Deletes incorrect chart entry.	○	○
Ability to add perio charting.	○	○
Makes patient appointment.	○	○
Cancels appointment.	○	○
Moves appointment to alternate date.	○	○
Successfully writes a prescription for a patient.	○	○
Updates the status of a patient.	○	○

Grade: _____   Student's Initials _____   Instructor's Initials _____

EVALUATION OF CHAPTER KNOWLEDGE CHECKLIST

Practice Management

Knowledge	Successful	Needs Assistance
Demonstrates entering a new employer.	○	○
Demonstrates adding new insurance for patient.	○	○
Demonstrates use of drop-down arrows to save time.	○	○
Creates quick letter.	○	○
Creates letter.	○	○
Creates postcard mailing.	○	○
Produces referral report.	○	○
Produces production report.	○	○
Explains how to view items prior to printing.	○	○
Shows how to edit an existing letter.	○	○
Accesses and navigates the patient ledger.	○	○
Locates specific icons quickly.	○	○
Produces patient walkout statement.	○	○

Grade: _____   Student's Initials _____   Instructor's Initials _____

Workbook Answer Key

Introduction to the Dental Profession

Multiple Choice

1. d   2. c   3. b   4. c   5. b   6. c   7. c

8. b   9. a   10. d

Matching

Match the individual with his contribution.

1. c   2. d   3. b   4. g   5. a   6. e   7. f

Critical Thinking

1. Education, efficiency, loyalty, and service.

2. a. Opportunities in continuing education, access to professional liability insurance, and the ADAA publication, *The Dental Assistant: Journal of the ADAA.*

    b. http://www.dentalassistant.org

    c. Membership offers dental assistants a voice in national affairs affecting the profession, and opportunities for interaction with professional peers.

3. a. 1790   b. 1760–1819   c. 1844   d. 1871   e. 1950

    f. 1960   g. 1938   h. 1982   i. 1832   j. 1997

    k. 1907   l. 1989   m. 1895

Case Study 1

1. She will likely see her general dentist first, if possible. X-rays may be necessary in order to reveal an impacted wisdom tooth/third molar. Periodic eruption is normal at this age. In Gwen's case, the x-ray reveals that it will not get better.

2. Oral maxillofacial surgeon.

Case Study 2

1. Periodontist—gum and bone loss.

2. Endodontist—decay has infected both the pulp canal and root/apex of the anterior tooth.

3. Oral and maxillofacial surgeon—impacted third molar.

4. Oral pathologist—lesion unknown in general dentistry.

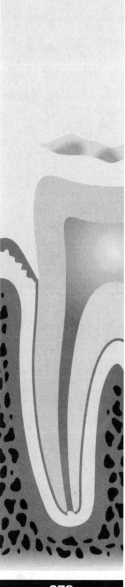

Psychology, Communication, and Multicultural Interaction

True or False

1. a

2. b. The dental assistant should be observant of a patient's behavior and needs, and tailor the methods used to communicate and treat that patient to meet those needs.

3. a

4. b. The kinesthetic channel involves using a caring or procedural touch when communicating with the patient.

5. b. A paradigm is an acquired belief system that a person establishes through various life experiences.

Multiple Choice

1. b	2. b	3. b	4. a	5. a	6. d	7. a

8. b	9. b	10. d

Matching

Match each term with the appropriate definition.

1. d	2. c	3. a	4. b

Communication consists of five major process components. Match each term with its process.

5. c	6. d	7. a	8. e	9. b

Critical Thinking

1. Nonverbal. The dental assistant needs to acknowledge what was observed. He or she can ask the patient if he is alright and if he is in pain or needs anything. The dental assistant can provide a caring or procedural touch to try to calm the patient.

2. Since the dental assistant is speaking to the patient to explain how to floss, that message is being delivered via verbal communication through the auditory channel. The dental assistant is also providing a demonstration of the technique that delivers the message through the visual channel of communication. Often more than one channel can be used to appropriately convey a message.

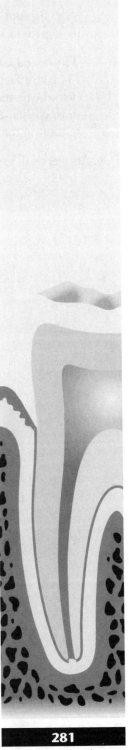

3. Active listening is crucial. The receiver encodes the message and responds, which may require analysis and interpretation of information. It may be necessary to repeat the content back to the dentist for clarity. When the mind wanders, listening stops. Eliminate barriers that diminish the ability to listen.

4. Listening is critical in the dental office. The telephone is where the patient forms his or her first impression of the dental office team. Thus, the telephone is lifeline of the office. The dental assistant should be empathetic to the patient's situation. The dental assistant should:

    * Listen for inflections in the patient's voice as to urgency.

    * Ask appropriate questions to ensure that the message being received and sent is accurate.

    * Promptly address the patient's need to be seen by scheduling an appointment to meet the patient's needs.

5. The dental assistant should be able to recognize common defense mechanisms and work with the patient to make effective communication possible. Understanding and recognizing patients' defense mechanisms help the dental team get to the truth. In addition to listening intently to verbal messages, dental assistants must constantly observe nonverbal behaviors and look for cues. Patients must have the assistant's full attention so that communication has every opportunity to succeed.

6. Answers will vary but should be good descriptions relevant to each of Maslow's hierarchy levels.

Ethics, Jurisprudence, and the Health Information Portability and Accountability Act

True or False

1. a   2. a   3. b   4. a   5. a

Multiple Choice

1. c   2. d   3. b   4. b   5. a   6. c   7. d

8. a   9. b   10. c   11. d   12. c   13. b   14. d

15. c   16. d   17. c   18. c   19. c   20. a   21. c

22. a   23. d   24. b   25. b

Matching

Match each word or term with its definition.

1. c   2. a   3. d   4. b

Critical Thinking

HIPAA and Compliance

1. a. Enacted to establish safeguards for health care transactions transmitted electronically.

    b. Designed to protect patient rights.

    c. Every dental office that chooses to transmit transactions electronically falls under HIPAA. By statute, it applies to all direct and indirect providers of health care services and supplies.

Business Associates

2. a. The dental office must have contracts with any business associates (including indirect providers or business associates that include maintenance services) that will be able to access individuals' PHI.

    b. Protected Health Information (PHI). HIPAA is safeguarding the PHI. It covers the individual or gives a reasonable basis in identifying the individual. The dental office must protect all patient records.

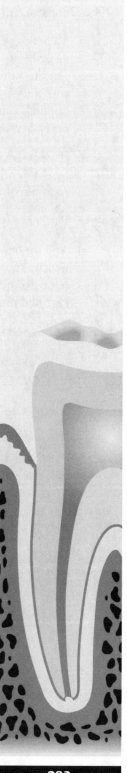

283

   c. Protection of patients' names, telephone numbers, fax numbers, e-mail addresses, social security numbers, student identification numbers, photographs, oral health information, birth dates, appointment dates, and any geographical identifier smaller than the state. Also, past, present, or future physical or mental health treatment.

   d. Doors must be locked when patient records are left unattended. Records cannot be left out for other to see. Day Sheets that show the daily schedule with patients' names and services cannot be left out for others to see.

The Dentist, Dental Assistant, and the Law

3. a. A contract can be expressed or implied. An expressed contract is written or verbally agreed upon. It describes specifically what each party in the contract will do. An implied contract is implemented by actions, not words. Most of the dentist/patient contracts are implied. If a patient comes to the dentist with a toothache and the dentist checks the area and requests that a radiograph be taken, this is an implied contract because it exists due to the circumstances. The law says that the dentist does what is necessary and what the patient would have requested had there been an expressed contract.

   b. Patient discharges the dentist or fails to return to the office. Patient fails to follow instructions given by the dentist. Dentist formally withdraws from patient care. Patient no longer needs treatment /all requirements agreed upon have been met.

   c. Patient fails to follow instructions from the dentist.

   d. Any time the patient fails to respond to or follow instructions of the dentist, the contract between the dentist and the patient is broken. When the patient discharges the dentist, the dentist should send a letter to the patient to confirm and document the termination of the contract. Letter should be sent certified mail.

Transactions and Code Sets, including Table 3.1

4. a. The first codes were set in 1969. Initially revised every 5 years, and now every 2 years. The latest revision was released in 2011.

   b. Centers for Medicare and Medicaid (CMS) is the enforcement authority.

   c. The Office for Civil Rights (ORC) is the enforcement authority for the privacy rule. The Centers for Medicare and Medicaid (CMS) is the enforcement authority for the transactions, code sets, identifiers, and security.

Oral Health and Preventive Techniques

True or False

1. a	2. b	3. a	4. a	5. a	6. a	7. b
8. b	9. b	10. a				

Multiple Choice

1. d	2. d	3. c	4. c	5. c	6. d	7. d
8. c	9. b	10. d	11. d	12. d	13. b	14. d
15. d						

Matching

Patient motivation is critical for the successful prevention of dental disease. Match the age characteristic with the general characteristics of that group.

1. c	2. a	3. b	4. e	5. d

Following are the various toothbrushing techniques and methods of use. Match the correct toothbrushing technique with its descriptive method.

6. c	7. d	8. e	9. b	10. a

Match the term with the best definition.

11. b	12. a	13. d	14. c

Match the term with the best definition.

15. c	16. a	17. e	18. b	19. d

Critical Thinking

1. Patients can use yarn in place of floss or a disposable elastomeric cleaning appliance and interproximal brushes.

2. A plastic scaler is used in the dental office to thoroughly clean teeth and remove all calculus.

3. Nausea is common in pregnancy. Nausea may cause regurgitation, during which teeth surfaces are repeatedly exposed to stomach acid. Patients need to be warned about potential damage to their teeth from repetitive exposure of teeth to stomach acid.

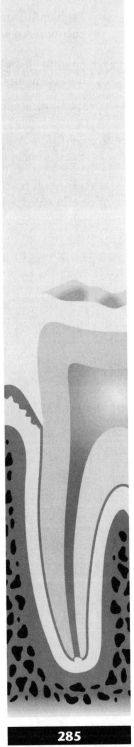

285

4. Suggestions could include eliminating toothpaste and identifying times of day when the pregnant patient is less nauseated.

Case Study

1. Listen to the patient and the concerns of the patient. Clearly communicate methods that will address those concerns and help to create better oral health. For example, if appearance is a concern communicate good oral hygiene and the affect it has on appearance. Answer all questions truthfully.

2. Asking questions of the patient and listening to the responses and the care the patient currently takes in her oral health. Be aware of the patient's body language and what it may be suggesting about her attitude.

3. Problem solving, being able to listen to the patients concerns and applying knowledge of the conditions encountered and addressing those issues with the patient based upon her needs and concerns.

4. Examine patient's dexterity and knowledge about proper technique, demonstrate proper technique, explain how to incorporate better oral health into her lifestyle.

5. Brushing and flossing regularly.

6. Dental decay (caries) equation:
   Sugar + plaque = acid + tooth = decay

Discuss foods that are typically eaten and how to care for the teeth after the foods are consumed or avoidance of certain types of carious foods.

Nutrition

True or False

1. a	2. a	3. a	4. b	5. b	6. b	7. a

8. a	9. b	10. a

Multiple Choice

1. a	2. b	3. a	4. d	5. c	6. a	7. b

8. a	9. d	10. d

Matching

Match the vitamin with how the body uses it.

1. b	2. d	3. a	4. c

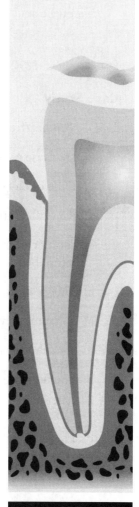

Critical Thinking

1. Water-soluble vitamins and fat-soluble vitamins.

2.

Carotene or retinol	Vitamin A	Fat-soluble	Whole milk/green leafy vegetables	Healthy skin
Thiamin	Vitamin B_1	Water-soluble	Eggs/fish/legumes	Coenzyme in oxidation of glucose
Riboflavin	Vitamin B_2	Water-soluble	Milk, cereals	Aids in release of energy
Pyridoxine	Vitamin B_6	Water-soluble	Whole grain/cereals	Antibody production
	Vitamin B_{12}	Water-soluble	Seafood/meat/eggs	Synthesis of red blood cells
Ascorbic acid	Vitamin C	Water-soluble	All citrus/broccoli	Healing wounds
Cholecalciferol	Vitamin D	Fat-soluble	Eggs/liver/fortified milk	Bone growth/tooth development
Alphatocopherol	Vitamin E	Fat-soluble	Margarine/salad dressing	Antioxidants
	Vitamin K	Fat-soluble	Cabbage/egg yolk/liver	Blood clotting
Folic acid	Folacin	Water-soluble	Spinach/asparagus/kidney beans	Synthesis of red blood cells
Nicotinic acid	Niacin	Water-soluble	Fish/poultry/eggs	Prevents gastrointestinal and nervous system problems

Case Study

1. a. Number/frequency of times that cariogenic foods are eaten.

   b. Are these cariogenic foods eaten with other foods?

   c. Time of day eaten.

   d. How often are the teeth exposed to cariogenic food? Complete calculation.

2. a. Eating cariogenic food with other foods may help neutralize acid. Cariogenic foods should not be eaten before bedtime.

   b. Choose carbohydrates that will not remain on the teeth a long time. Consume more fruit and grains.

3. a. Calcium. Development of bones and teeth.

   b. Phosphorus. Maintain pH balance in blood.

4. a. The body's needs are increased for mother and baby.

   b. To maintain an adequate diet to avoid malnutrition in mother and baby.

   c. The essential nutrients maintain the body's metabolism and balance the energy used daily.

5. Supplemental nutrients include vitamins and minerals.

General Anatomy and Physiology

True or False

1. a	2. a	3. a	4. b	5. b	6. b	7. a
8. b	9. a	10. a				

Multiple Choice

1. d	2. d	3. b	4. d	5. a	6. d	7. d
8. d	9. b	10. b	11. d	12. d	13. a	14. b
15. a	16. d	17. b	18. a	19. d	20. b	21. d
22. a	23. b	24. a	25. b	26. c	27. d	28. a
29. b	30. a	31. d	32. d	33. d	34. d	35. b

Matching

Identify each muscle with the matching muscle characteristic.

1. c	2. a	3. d	4. b

Critical Thinking

1. Type of muscle by description:

    Striated

    Cardiac

    Smooth

2. Excitability and irritability.

3. Muscle characteristic by description:

    Extensibility

    Muscle tone

    Isometric contraction

    Isotonic contraction

4. Strain, sprain, cramp, inflammation, and spasm.

5. If a muscle is not used, it deteriorates.

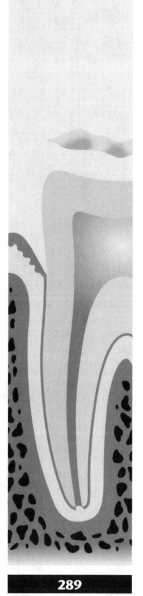

Case Study 1

1. MS (multiple sclerosis) is a disease.

2. MS usually is diagnosed in people aged 20 to 40 years.

3. The central nervous system is affected. The disease destroys the myelin sheath of neurons.

4. Impulses cannot transmit to their destination. Therefore their dental responses will be slower—depending on the degree or stage of MS.

Case Study 2

1. Endocrine and reproductive systems.

2. The endocrine system generally controls the body's growth, protects the body in stressful situations, regulates utilization of calcium, aids in regulating the body's water balance, and produces insulin, which aids in the transport of glucose into the cells.

3. See Table 6-5 for major glands of the endocrine system.

4. The main function of the reproductive system in men and women is reproduction, or the creation of life.

5. Dental treatment may need to be altered depending on the stage of pregnancy.

Head and Neck Anatomy

True or False

1. a   2. b   3. b   4. b   5. a   6. a

7. b   8. a.   9. a   10. b

Multiple Choice

1. a   2. a   3. d   4. b   5. a   6. d   7. a

8. d   9. b   10. b   11. a   12. b   13. b   14. b

15. c   16. a   17. c   18. b   19. b   20. b   21. c

22. d   23. d   24. a   25. b   26. a   27. b   28. d

29. d   30. b   31. a   32. d   33. a   34. b   35. d

36. d   37. d   38. a   39. b   40. d

Matching

Match the landmarks with the correct terms.

1. b   2. d   3. e   4. c   5. a

Match each landmark in the palatal area of the oral cavity with the correct description.

6. e   7. d   8. b   9. c   10. a

Match the nerve branch with its service.

11. d   12. a   13. b   14. c

Landmarks of palatal and oral pharynx area.

15. b   16. c   17. d   18. a

Match the term with the region of the tongue description.

19. b   20. a   21. d   22. c

Critical Thinking

1. Ala of the nose: wing of the nose or outer edge of the nostril. Naso-labial groove: groove from the ala of the nose to the corners of the mouth. Philtrum: shallow, V-shaped depression between the bottom of the nose and the middle of the upper lip.

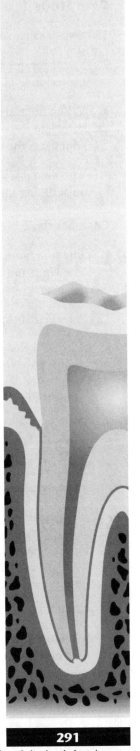

291

2. Labial commissures: the corners of the mouth.

3. Uvula: projection that extends off the back of the soft palate. Anterior tonsillar pillars: folds of tissue extending horizontally from the uvula to the base of the tongue; also known as palatoglossal arches. Posterior tonsillar pillars: found farther back in the throat; also known as palatopharyngeal arches. Palatine tonsils: situated between the two sets of pillars is a depressed area and the location of this tonsil; often marked with deep grooves and are red and inflamed due to infection. Fauces: space in the back of the oral cavity where food passes into the pharynx.

4. Torus mandibularis.

Case Study 1

1. Sweet, salty, sour, and bitter.

2. Sweet receptors are located on the tip of the tongue, salty on the anterior side of the tongue, sour on the posterior sides of the tongue, and bitter in the center posterior section of the tongue.

3. When the taste bud is stimulated with various chemicals, receptors carry taste impulses to the brain. To stimulate the sense of taste, substances (food) must be mixed with liquid to form a solution. The solution stimulates the receptors to generate one or a combination of the four taste sensations.

4. The dental assistant should be aware that certain drugs cause patients to lose their sense of taste. Further questioning may be necessary to evaluate this response.

Case Study 2

1. The function of saliva is to moisten and lubricate the oral cavity and to moisten food, aiding in mastication (chewing) and swallowing of food. Saliva also initiates the digestion of starches and helps to regulate water balance.

2. Parotid glands, submandibular glands, and sublingual glands.

3. Saliva is a clear fluid. Viscosity may vary according to fluid in the saliva. Effects depend on an individual's chemical makeup, diet, and medications.

4. Dry mouth is caused by an abnormal reduction in the amount of saliva secretion.

5. Diseases that may be related to dry mouth include diabetes. Dry mouth may also result from radiation or chemotherapy.

6. The dental assistant's response to the patient may be informing her or him of products that ameliorate dry mouth symptoms. Further assessment may be necessary to identify individual needs.

Case Study 3

1. Parotid glands.

2. Swelling and tenderness.

3. Children aged 5 to 15 are the most commonly affected.

4. Sometimes the salivary glands develop crystallizations or stones. When these stones try to leave the glands, they block the ducts. Swelling immediately occurs and the stones must be surgically removed.

Labeling

Muscles of mastication.

1. f	2. d	3. e	4. g	5. c	6. b	7. a

Muscles of facial expression.

8. a	9. d	10. f	11. e	12. c

Maxillary arch nerves.

13. c	14. a	15. d	16. h	17. l	18. e	19. k	20. j
21. f	22. i	23. g	24. b				

Mandibular nerves.

25. a	26. k	27. d	28. g and i	29. b	30. e	31. h and j
32. f	33. c					

Embryology and Histology

Multiple Choice

1. d	2. c	3. b	4. c	5. a	6. d	7. b
8. b	9. c	10. c	11. b	12. d	13. b	14. c
15. d	16. a	17. d	18. d	19. b	20. d	21. b
22. c	23. c	24. c	25. a	26. b	27. c	28. a
29. d	30. b	31. d	32. d	33. b	34. d	35. d
36. a						

Matching

Identify the types of dentin and their functions.

1. c	2. e	3. d	4. b	5. a

Match the terms for pregnancy phases by time period.

6. c	7. a	8. b

Critical Thinking

1. a. A root canal therapy may be necessary. The pulp tissue is removed and the tooth becomes nonvital.

   b. If the pulp is damaged due to an injury, the tissue may become inflamed, causing pulpitis. The pressure increases and cannot escape. The structures of the tooth form a hard encasement and, when the tooth becomes inflamed it cause a great deal of pressure and discomfort. The patient may need to have root canal therapy, which opens the pulp and releases the pressure.

   c. The use of water-cooled handpieces prevents overheating of the pulp during dental treatment.

   d. Pulp stones—calcified masses of dentin—are sometimes in the pulp tissue. They can be attached or unattached to the pulpal wall. They are quite common and normally cause a problem only if root canal therapy is necessary.

2. a. Dental hypersensitivity, dentin exposed. This may be very painful for the patient. In some individuals, the enamel and cementum do not come together at the cementoenamel junction (CEJ), leaving exposed dentin, which results in dentinal hypersensitivity.

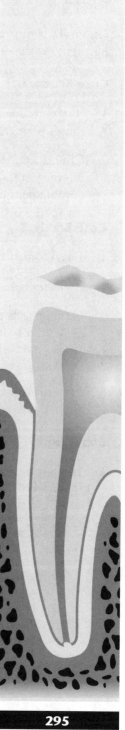

b. Next, in the case of gingival recession, the cementum may become exposed. The cementum is very thin at the cementoenamel junction and can quickly wear away.

3. a. Alveolar bone: periodontal ligament and gingival fiber group.

b. Alveolar bone: Periodontal disease can cause the loss of bone. The bone does not regenerate and the diseased tissue must be removed. The bone is stimulated from mastication and speech. If the teeth are removed, this stimulation is lost and the bone can resorb. The bone supports the teeth and the teeth support the bone.

Periodontal ligament: Occlusal trauma does not cause periodontal disease but can accelerate existing disease. Chronic periodontal disease causes the fiber groups to become disorganized and lose attachment due to resorption.

Gingival fiber group: The fiber group that is retained the longest during periodontal disease is the interdental ligament. As the disease progresses, this ligament reattaches itself in a more apical manner.

Case Study 1

1. If tetracycline is taken as an antibiotic during the formation of dentin, it binds chemically to the dentin and causes permanent yellow staining.

2. Clinical considerations: Dentin is what gives the translucent enamel its underlying yellow hue. Drug interaction such as an antibiotic tetracycline taken during the formation of dentin can disrupt the development process.

Case Study 2

1. Loss of nutritional support during the apposition stage.

2. Apposition stage.

3. Calcium salts and other minerals are deposited in the formed tooth. The tissues—enamel, dentin, and cementum—are formed in layers.

4. Yes.

5. Fluoride can aid in strengthening the enamel to prevent demineralization. Fluoride can be ingested or applied topically.

Labeling

For labeling answers, see the following figures in the textbook (in this order): 8–4, 8–5, 8–13, 8–17, 8–19, 8–15, and 8–16.

Tooth Morphology

True or False

1. a   2. a   3. a   4. b   5. a

Multiple Choice

1. c   2. b   3. c   4. b   5. b   6. b   7. b

8. c   9. d   10. a   11. c   12. b

Matching

Match each term with its definition.

1. b   2. d   3. a   4. c

Match the terms with the deciduous teeth in the diagram.

5. b   6. e   7. a   8. c   9. d

Critical Thinking

1. See Figure 9-4 in the textbook.
2. Refer to Table 9-1 in the textbook.

Case Study 1

1. Maxillary

   a. Deciduous canine: 5

   b. Deciduous lateral incisor: 3

   c. Deciduous first molar: 7

   d. Deciduous second molar: 9

   e. Permanent central incisor: 1

   f. Permanent lateral incisor: 2

   g. Permanent first molar: 10

   h. Permanent first premolar: 6

   i. Permanent second molar: 11

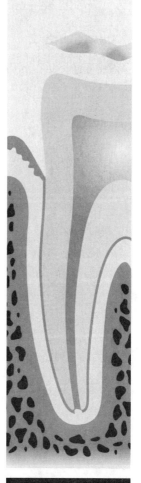

     j. Permanent second premolar: 8

     k. Permanent canine: 4

     Mandibular

     a. Deciduous canine: 4

     b. Deciduous first molar: 5

     c. Deciduous second molar: 7

     d. Permanent canine: 3

     e. Permanent central incisor: 1

     f. Permanent lateral incisor: 2

     g. Permanent first molar: 9

     h. Permanent first premolar: 6

     i. Permanent second molar: 10

     j. Permanent second premolar: 8

2. This will be the permanent second premolar.

3. Either maxillary or mandibular would be age 11 to 12. In order of permanent teeth eruption, the maxillary would be number 5, and, if mandibular, it would be number 6.

Case Study 2

See Table 9-2 in the textbook.

Microbiology

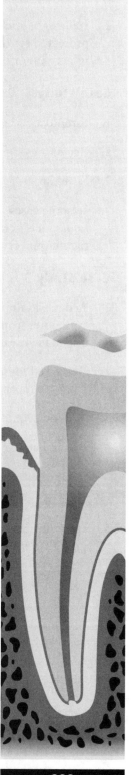

True or False

1. b	2. a	3. b	4. b	5. a	6. b	7. a
8. a	9. b	10. a				

Multiple Choice

1. b	2. a	3. c	4. d	5. b	6. b	7. a
8. b	9. d	10. a	11. b	12. c	13. a	14. b
15. d	16. d	17. c	18. c	19. b	20. c	21. d
22. b	23. d	24. c	25. d	26. c	27. b	28. b
29. b	30. c	31. b	32. b	33. a	34. d	35. b
36. b	37. c	38. c	39. d	40. b	41. d	42. c
43. d	44. c					

Matching

Match each important person with his contribution to microbiology.

1. b   2. c   3. a

Match each type of microorganism with disease or symptoms.

4. d   5. c   6. b   7. a

Match each of the following diseases of major concern to the dental assistant with its respective infection.

8. c   9. d   10. a   11. b

Critical Thinking

1. Cohn described the life cycle of *Bacillus* and showed that bacteria could go into an endospore state upon being boiled (encountering extremely negative environmental conditions), and would not be killed. In the modern dental office, tests ensure that endospores have been destroyed during the sterilization process.

2. Creating vaccines.

3. People around age 60. Symptoms include rapidly progressing dementia, memory loss, speech impairment, involuntary jerky movements, weakness, blindness, and then coma. The disease progresses rapidly, and is fatal due to neurological degeneration.

4. Ingestion of contaminated water or food.

Case Study 1

1. Hepatitis A, B, C, D, and E.

2. Injuries or sticks with sharp objects contaminated with blood or body fluid; multiple sexual partners, unprotected sex (homosexual, bisexual, or heterosexual); sharing contaminated needles; and exposure to nonintact skin or open wound with contaminated blood or body fluid.

Case Study 2

1. Streptococci.

2. Bacteria elongate and divide into two separate cells, and then continuously repeat this cycle.

3. Sore throat, fever, and general malaise.

4. In some cases, toxins released by the bacteria can cause a rash, and can lead to scarlet fever. *Streptococcus mutans* has been found to cause dental caries and endocarditis. The same group of bacteria can give rise to pneumonia or rheumatic fever.

Case Study 3

1. Acquired immunity occurs as a result of exposure to a pathogen. Passive acquired immunity occurs when antibodies from another individual are injected into an individual, giving protection to the individual from a specific disease.

2. Borrowed immunity is also called passive acquired immunity. A fetus obtains temporary passive immunity from the mother through the placenta.

3. Natural acquired immunity and artificial acquired immunity.

4. Natural acquired immunity occurs when an individual has had a disease, the body has manufactured antibodies to the disease, and the person has recovered from the disease. Normally the individual is then immune to the disease. Artificial acquired immunity occurs when the individual is vaccinated with a specific antigen.

5. If the antigen causes an allergic response, it is called an allergen. Individuals more sensitive to certain allergens than most are called hypersensitive. In a severe case, a person's antigen-antibody stimulates a massive secretion of histamine. This severe reaction, called anaphylactic shock, is sometimes fatal.

CHAPTER 11

Infection Control

True or False

1. a	2. a	3. a	4. b	5. a	6. a	7. a
8. b	9. b	10. b				

Multiple Choice

1. d	2. a	3. b	4. a	5. b	6. d	7. b
8. a	9. c	10. a	11. d	12. c	13. b	14. d
15. a	16. d	17. b	18. c	19. d	20. a	21. c
22. d	23. a	24. b	25. d	26. c	27. c	28. c
29. c	30. b	31. b	32. b	33. a	34. a	35. d
36. d	37. c	38. a	39. b	40. b		

Matching

Match the following standards with the protection that they provide.

1. b	2. c	3. d	4. a

Match the glove with its designated use.

5. d	6. a	7. b	8. c

Match the sterilization method with its use.

9. c	10. a	11. d	12. b

Critical Thinking

1. Government agencies (such as OSHA) and licensing boards that have the authority to enforce compliance.

2. Dentists may be fined, lose their licenses to practice dentistry, or face imprisonment.

3. Can be made by anyone, and no authority for enforcement is mandated.

4. Other potentially infectious materials. Employers must protect their employees not only from exposure to blood but also from OPIM during the time when employees are at work.

5. Employees (full-time, part-time, and temporary) who fall into categories 1 and/or 2, where tasks involve exposure to blood, body fluid such as saliva, and/or body

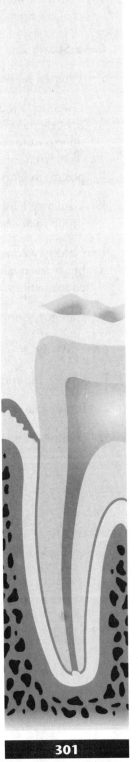

tissues, must have training. Training must be provided at no cost to the dental assistant employee. Training must be given—before placement in a position where bloodborne pathogens are a factor—to all new employees and to all employees reclassifying into these positions.

Case Study 1

1. Occupational Safety and Health Administration (OSHA).

2. OSHA Bloodborne Pathogens Standard.

3. Provide communication on biohazards. Establish standards for handling and disposal of hazardous waste. (Follow Step 3 of the OSHA Written Exposure Plan.)

Case Study 2

1. Written exposure plan.

2. Category 1 includes all tasks that involve exposure to blood, body fluids such as saliva, or body tissues (dentists, dental assistant, dental hygienist, and laboratory technician). Category 2 includes all tasks that involve no exposure to blood, body fluids such as saliva, or body tissues, but occasionally may involve unplanned tasks from category 1 (receptionist, coordinating assistant). Category 3 includes all tasks that involve no exposure to blood, body fluids such as saliva, or body tissues (accountant, insurance assistant).

3. Category 1 includes tasks that involve exposure to blood, body fluids such as saliva, and body tissues. (This group includes dentist, dental assistant, dental hygienist, and dental laboratory technician.)

4. Category 2 includes all tasks that involve no exposure to blood, body fluids such as saliva, or body tissues, but occasionally may involve unplanned tasks from Category 1. (This group includes the receptionist, coordinating assistant, and so on.)

5. Category 3 includes all tasks that involve no exposure to blood, body fluids such as saliva, or body tissues

Case Study 3

1. Direct, indirect, and inhalation/aerosol.

2. Immunization, hepatitis B series.

3. Handwashing.

Management of Hazardous Materials

Multiple Choice

1. d	2. b	3. a	4. d	5. b	6. d	7. c
8. d	9. c	10. a	11. b	12. d	13. b	14. c
15. c	16. b	17. d	18. b	19. c		

Matching

Match the fluid with its excretion.

1. c	2. d	3. e	4. a	5. b

Match the color with its hazard type/warning.

6. b	7. d	8. a	9. c

Critical Thinking

1. Under the Needlestick Safety and Prevention Act, OSHA guidelines are as follows: no recapping, breaking, or bending of needles upon completing a procedure. Contaminated sharps and needles must be placed immediately in a labeled, leakproof, puncture-resistant container upon procedure completion.

2. Required whenever there is potential for splashing, spraying, or splattering to the eyes or mucous membranes. Prescription glasses may be fitted with solid-side shields.

3. See flowchart for occupational exposure to bloodborne pathogens (Figure 12-4 in textbook).

Case Study 1

1. Understanding OSHA Bloodborne/Hazardous Materials Standards and then applying them are the responsibility of each dental team member. Under the Information and Training segment, training occurs shortly after employment of team member, annually, and when a new product is introduced.

2. Yes. On the MSDS Form X. Special Precautions. Example: Precaution to be taken in handling and storing: avoid contact with eyes.

3. Yes. Also the MSDS Form IX, Protection Information/Control Measures. Example: Eye: Safety glasses; Gloves: Not required.

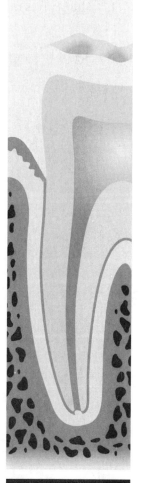

4. Each offce must have a manual of material safety data sheets that is alphabetized, indexed, and available to all employees. The location of the manual will vary based upon office practice; be sure to know where the log is kept in any practice you work in.

5. Yes. Training records are kept for 3 years from date of training. Employees must have a certifcate available or in their personnel file that shows they have had the proper training. A log is required to include training as specified in the written plan.

Case Study 2

1. The product would have a chemical warning label. Labeling and material safety data sheets (MSDSs) also provide the manufacturer's product labeling instructions as well. Data sheets are stored in the office MSDS manual.

2. Red—fire hazard; yellow—reactivity; blue—health hazard; white—PPE.

3. Red—flammable liquid; yellow—may react if mixed with water; blue—harmful if inhaled; white—goggles, gloves, mask.

Case Study 3

1. Gloves must be worn whenever hands have contact with blood, OPIMs, mucous membranes, non-intact skin, or contaminated surfaces/items, or when performing vascular access procedures (phlebotomy).

2. Vinyl or latex for general use. Utility gloves for surface disinfection. Puncture-resistant gloves for handling sharps (e.g., central supply).

3. Alternatives must be available if the employee has allergic reactions (e.g., powderless gloves).

Preparation for Patient Care

True or False

1. a   2. b   3. b   4. b   5. b

Multiple Choice

1. b   2. d   3. a   4. b   5. b   6. d   7. c

8. d   9. a   10. d   11. c   12. b   13. d   14. c

15. b   16. b   17. d   18. c   19. d   20. b   21. d

22. b   23. a   24. c   25. b

Matching

Match the term with its definition.

1. b   2. d   3. a   4. c

Match the term with the best definition.

5. d   6. c   7. b   8. a

Match the term with the best definition.

9. b   10. c   11. d   12. a

Match the term with the best definition.

13. b   14. e   15. d   16. a   17. c

Critical Thinking

1. a. Is the personal information correct (e.g., emergency contact, physician name/phone number)?

   b. Past surgeries.

   c. Allergies to latex, antibiotics.

   d. Medical concerns, such as diabetes, heart condition.

   e. Any drugs taken recently or currently.

2. Clinical observation and clinical evaluation.

3. a. Smile line (where the lips are when the patient smiles).

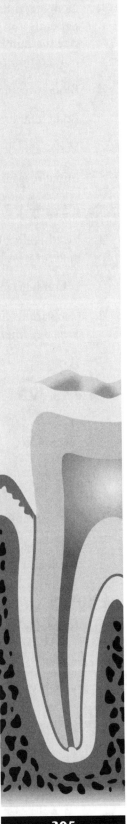

b. Vermilion border (the line around the lips).

c. Commissures (the corners of the lips).

Case Study 1

1. "Palpate, inflate, obliterate, deflate" method. While listening with the stethoscope, place the cuff on the patient's arm and palpate the radial pulse. Slowly inflate the cuff just until the pulse is obliterated, memorize the number, and release the pressure in the bulb. Add 30 mmHg to the number representing the pulse obliteration point. Wait one minute; then, using the above figure, proceed to take the blood pressure.

2. Blood pressure.

3. Body temperature, pulse, respiration, blood pressure.

4. Yes.

5. Initial measurements of vital signs.

Case Study 2

1. Yes. Likely due to completing an hour of exercise at a gym before the appointment. The rush of excitement of possibly being late for his appointment could also contribute.

2. Fahrenheit: range 96.0–99.5, average 98.6. Celsius: range 35.5–37.5, average 37.0.

3. Can vary from person to person and at different times of the day. Body temperature may be elevated after exercise, emotional excitement, or eating or drinking something hot.

4. Yes.

Case Study 3

1. Normal pulse rate for adults is 60 to 90 beats per minute. Normal pulse rate for children is 90 to 120 beats per minute.

2. Normal respiration rate in adults is 12 to 18 respirations per minute. Normal respiration rate in children is 20 to 40 respirations per minute.

3. Normal range in Fahrenheit is 99.5–96.0, average 98.6. Celsius

4. Normal blood pressure readings: child 10 years of age 100/66; adolescent 16 years of age 118/76; adult systolic below 140, diastolic below 90.

Labeling

1. Vermilion border

2. Commissures of the lip

3. Smile line

Dental Charting

True or False

1. a	2. a	3. b	4. b	5. a	6. a	7. b
8. b	9. a	10. b				

Multiple Choice

1. a	2. b	3. d	4. d	5. c	6. c	7. d
8. b	9. d	10. a	11. b	12. b	13. c	14. d
15. d	16. c	17. c	18. c	19. b	20. a	21.d
22. d	23. c	24. b	25. d	26. d	27. d	28. b
29. d	30. b					

Matching

Match the cavity classification with the surface area(s).

1. d	2. a	3. b	4. e	5. c

Match the system with its corresponding coding.

6. c	7. a	8. b

Match the corresponding charting symbols.

9. e	10. d	11. b	12. a	13. c

Critical Thinking

1.　a. In blue, MO; in red, DO.

　　b. Classification II.

2.　a. Between 29 and 30.

　　b. #19.

　　c. #14.

　　d. #22–27.

3.　See Figure 14-3 in textbook.

4.　Between 4/5, 7/8, and 11/12.

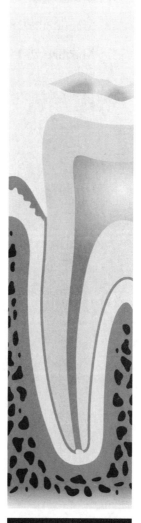

Case Study 1

1. Between 4 and 5, 13 and 14, and 19 and 20.

2. Between 1 and 2 = 6 mm, between 2 and 3 = 4 mm, between 14 and 15 = 6 mm, and between 17 and 18 = 6 mm.

3. #7.

4. #30.

5. # 2, #14, and #18.

Case Study 2

1. C–H and M–R.

2. A–B, I–J, K–L, and S–T.

3. 3, 6–11, 14, 19, 22–27, and 30.

4. 1–2, 4–5, 12–13, 15–16, 17–18, 20–21, 28–29, and 31–32.

Case Study 3

1. Maxillary 1–16, and mandibular 17–21 and 28–32.

2. Mandibular 28–31 and 18–21

3. Maxillary 2–15.

Pharmacology

Multiple Choice

1. c	2. b	3. d	4. c	5. b	6. a	7. d
8. c	9. b	10. c	11. c	12. d	13. c	14. d
15. b	16. a	17. a	18. b	19. c	20. b	21. d
22. a	23. c	24. b	25. a			

Matching

Match each term with its definition.

1. d	2. e	3. a	4. b	5. c

Match each term with the best definition.

6. g	7. f

Match administration by route of injection.

8. c	9. d	10. b	11. a

Critical Thinking

1. a. a.c.: before meals.

    b. q.i.d.: four times a day.

    c. q.h.: every hour.

    d. q.4.h.: every four hours.

    e. p.c.: after meals.

2. Whether the prescription is to be filled with a brand-name drug or a generic drug.

3. a. Schedule I drugs have a high potential for abuse and no accepted medical use. Drugs include mescaline, marijuana, heroin, and LSD.

    b. Schedule II drugs have a high potential for abuse and are accepted for medical use. These drugs lead to physical and psychological dependence. Drugs include certain opioids (e.g., morphine, oxycodone), short-acting barbiturates (secobarbital), and amphetamines.

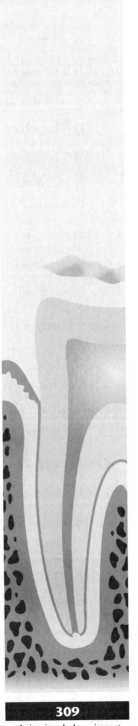

    c. Schedule III drugs have a lower potential for abuse and have accepted medical uses. These drugs are routinely prescribed in the dental office. They may lead to chemical dependency. Drugs in this schedule include intermediate-acting barbiturates, Tylenol III, and anabolic steroids.

    d. Schedule IV drugs have less potential for abuse and have acceptable medical uses. They have limited dependency. Drugs in this schedule include antidepressants, antianxiety drugs, and sedative drugs not included in the I, II, or III schedule of drugs.

    e. Schedule V drugs have the least potential for abuse. These drugs may contain a compound from other drug schedules. Also known as over-the-counter drugs, they include antidiarrheal medications, cough medicines, and analgesics.

4. (1) The heading includes the dentist's name, address, telephone number, and registration number.

    (2) The superscription includes the patient's name and address, and the date on which the prescription is written.

    (3) The subscription that includes the symbol Rx ("take thou").

    (4) The inscription that states the names and quantities of ingredients to be included in the medication.

    (5) The subscription that gives directions to the pharmacist for filling the prescription.

    (6) The signature (Sig): The directions the doctor gives to the patient.

    (7) Dentist's signature blanks: Where signed, indicates if a generic substitute is allowed or if the medication is to be dispensed as written.

    (8) REPETATUR 0, 1, 2, 3 p.r.n.: This is where the dentist indicates whether the prescription can be refilled.

    (9) = LABEL: Directions to the pharmacist to label the medication appropriately.

5. Intradermal injection

Case Study 1

1. Yes.

2. Alcohol, a depressant, has the opposite effect of a stimulant.

3. Under the legally defined level of intoxication, the patient can experience loss of judgment and coordination and exhibit slowed reactions and slurred speech.

Case Study 2

1. Yes. They are often prescribed as a prophylactic measure to prevent infection.

2. Resistance to antibiotics can develop. It often occurs when the user fails to take the antibiotic drug at the dosage directed and for as long as directed. The bacteria can return stronger and more resistant to the antibiotic.

3. Adverse side effects can include nausea, diarrhea, and an allergic rash, up to severe allergic reactions. Patients can also kill normal body flora, causing oral, intestinal, or vaginal candidiasis.

Case Study 3

1. Review of patient's medical and health history.

2. Drug types: anticholinergics, antidepressants, antihistamines, nitrates.

3. Antihistamine combined with the antidepressant; each will indicate possible side effects of dry mouth. Answers may vary.

Emergency Management

Multiple Choice

1. d	2. d	3. d	4. b	5. a	6. a	7. a
8. c	9. a	10. a	11. b	12. c	13. d	14. a
15. b	16. c	17. b	18. c	19. c	20. d	21. d
22. b	23. c	24. d	25. c	26. b	27. a	28. c
29. a	30. b	31. b	32. c	33. d	34. c	35. b
36. b	37. b	38. a	39. c	40. d		

Matching

Match the term with the definition.

1. d	2. c	3. e	4. a	5. b

Match the condition with its response.

6. c	7. d	8. e	9. b	10. a

Match the term with its characteristics.

11. d	12. c	13. b	14. a

Match the term with its condition.

15. e	16. c	17. a	18. b	19. d

Critical Thinking

1. Does the patient have difficulty moving? Do the patient's eyes respond to light? Is the patient's speech slurred? Does the patient indicate anxiety about the dental treatment?

2. A liver or heart transplant. The patient may have a pacemaker or be taking any number of drug therapies. Elderly patients in particular may be taking more than one drug. Some drugs taken prior to a dental treatment may interact with drugs given in treatment. Lengthy dental appointments may overtax the patient's ability to remain comfortable, thereby causing anxiety and stress that lead to an emergency situation.

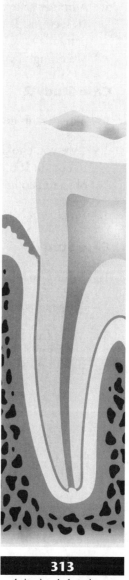

313

3. It is believed that valuable time was lost when trying to assess breathing and a pulse before beginning chest compressions. It is believed that this will increase survival rates of the cardiac events.

4. Both hyperventilation and syncope symptoms include rapid breathing and nervousness. Faintness is a hyperventilation symptom; in syncope, the patient at this point has lost consciousness. Treatment for hyperventilation: patient breathes into a paper bag and is helped to remain calm. For syncope, treatment consists of lowering the head to increase blood flow to the brain; may also require spirits of ammonia.

Case Study 1

1. Syncope is normally caused by some form of stress—emotional, physical, or both. The patient may feel dizzy, nauseated, or extremely weak before losing consciousness. The patient may appear pale and clammy, and breathes in shallow gasps.

2. When a patient experiences stress, the body reacts by pumping large amounts of blood to the arms and legs. Blood pools in the arms and legs and cerebral blood flow is diminished.

3. Talk to patients, assure them that everything is all right. Help them overcome the apprehension and fear of treatment.

4. Keep instruments, needles, and blood out of the patient's sight.

5. Administer oxygen and monitor vital signs. The patient will usually resume breathing in less than 10 seconds. If the patient becomes unconscious, break a vial of spirits of ammonia and pass it under the patient's nose. The strong odor of the ammonia causes the patient to quickly inhale, which stimulates breathing. Typically, the patient will revive within a couple of minutes.

Case Study 2

1. The person may begin choking and clutch the throat with hands.

2. "Are you choking?" The first action is to stop treatment, sit the patient upright, and encourage him or her to cough. If the patient cannot expel the object, the Heimlich maneuver should be performed until the object dislodges.

3. Amalgam, composite, cotton rolls, gauze, endodontic instruments, and impression material.

Case Study 3

1. Asthma may be triggered by an allergy to a substance.

2. Animal fur, house dust, pollens, tobacco smoke, feathers, food, and drugs.

3. More frequent in the morning, varying from slight breathlessness to respiratory failure.

4. Breathing should improve within 15 minutes.

CHAPTER 17

Introduction to the Dental Office and Basic Chairside Assisting

True or False

| 1. a | 2. a | 3. a | 4. b | 5. b | 6. a | 7. b |

| 8. a | 9. a | 10. a |

Multiple Choice

| 1. c | 2. d | 3. b | 4. d | 5. b | 6. a | 7. d |

| 8. c | 9. d | 10. c | 11. c | 12. b | 13. c | 14. d |

15. c

Matching

Match each classification of motion with its proper definition.

| 1. c | 2. e | 3. a | 4. b | 5. d |

Match the room to an office by its design and function.

| 6. d | 7. c | 8. a | 9. b |

Match the following activity zones for a right-handed operator with clock positions.

| 10. c | 11. d | 12. a | 13. b |

Critical Thinking

1. a. The stool is positioned 4 to 6 inches above the operator for good visibility.

   b. Position on the stool so that weight is distributed evenly over the seat.

   c. Front edge of the assistant's stool is even with the patient's mouth.

   d. Feet are resting on a flat ring or round base of stool or just above the casters, and thighs are parallel to the floor.

   e. Position as close as possible to the side of the patient.

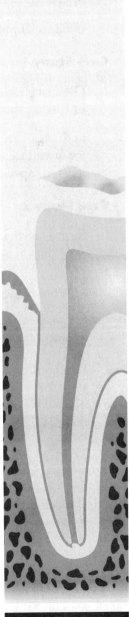

315

    f. Assistant's back is straight, with support in the lumbar region. Side support should extend around in front of the assistant. This extension supports the assistant when leaning forward. The side support adjusts to fit the level of the assistant's abdomen.

    g. After correctly positioning on the chair, the cabinet top or mobile cart is placed over the thighs as close as possible for convenience and efficiency.

2. Zones for a left-handed operatory:

    a. 12–5 o'clock, operating zone

    b. 8–10 o'clock, assistant zone

    c. 10–12 o'clock, static zone

    d. 5–8 o'clock, transfer zone

3. a. Class I motion involves only finger movement.

    b. Class II motion involves movement of the fingers and wrist.

    c. Class III motion involves finger, wrist, and elbow movement.

Case Study 1

1. Offer suggestions for the first dental appointment, such as bringing an interpreter, who may be a relative or friend (who would accompany the person anyway), or someone from a church or social agency.

2. Staff members may try to learn key words in the patient's language, and/or learn about the patient's country or culture. Pictures may be available to help the patient understand what is involved in a procedure and what to expect.

Case Study 2

1. Rear delivery system: equipment located behind the patient's head.

    Side delivery system: equipment designed to be on the dentist's side.

    Front delivery system: equipment designed so that it can be pulled over the patient's chest.

    Other, mobile carts: one cart each for the operator and the assistant with the appropriate access to either side of the dental chair.

2. Cart configuration types:

    Mobile instrumentation includes air-water syringe, oral evacuator, handpieces, and saliva ejector.

    One cart each may be used by the operator and by the assistant with the instrumentation on the appropriate side.

    Two carts, one on each side of the dental chair.

    Operator's cart is usually set up for two or three dental handpieces plus an air-water syringe.

    Assistant's cart is usually set up with the air-water syringe, saliva ejector, and high-volume evacuator (HVE). By design, carts should move easily, provide a workspace and some storage, and hold basic instruments.

3. Lights are attached to the dental chair or mounted to the ceiling.

    Both the operator and the assistant should be able to adjust the position of the light.

    Lights can be easier to move, more flexible, and direct less heat to the patient.

    Lights may be equipped with a control switch for high and low intensities, an on/off switch, and handles on both sides. The handles and switches are covered with barriers during each patient procedure. The barriers are changed before each patient.

Case Study 3

1. Operator stool:

    Adjustable height, so that the operator's feet can be flat on the floor and thighs parallel to the floor.

    Adjustable back rest, both vertically and horizontally, to provide support and comfort. The back rest should support the lumbar region of the operator's back.

    Comfortable seat, broad with firm padding, without seams or edges to restrict circulation in the legs and feet. Seat should also be covered with a material that is easy to clean.

    The stool should move easily and freely on four to five casters, even on floor with carpet.

    The stool should have a broad, heavy base to prevent tipping, especially during movement.

2. Dental assistant stool:

    The stool should adjust to various levels to accommodate the height of the assistant. The assistant is positioned 4 to 8 inches higher than the operator, with feet resting on the foot ring and thighs parallel to the floor.

    The stool back rest should provide support for the lumbar region and be easily adjustable. The extended arm should provide support of the abdomen or side areas. The arm moves easily into place and locks to stabilize the assistant when leaning or reaching.

    Comfortable seat, with the same criteria as the operator's stool.

    Chair should be designed to move freely. Usually, five casters are recommended to provide stability.

    Since the assistant is typically positioned higher than the operator, it is difficult to sit correctly on the stool and rest feet flat on the floor. The foot rest, which is easily adjusted, gives the assistant support so that good circulation is maintained. *All* parts of the assistant's stool should be easy to adjust.

Case Study 4

1. It is important that the reception room be pleasing and comfortable as well as neat and clean. The patient's first impression of the office is made in the reception area. Magazines should be current and appropriate for the dentist's clientele. The dental staff should tidy this room regularly.

2. The reception desk is usually adjacent to the reception room, so that patients can be greeted as they enter the office. This is the area where appointments are made, telephone calls are received, and patient records are updated and stored. The area may include counter space, desk space, adequate lighting, accessible filing system, and access to computer terminals and telecommunications systems.

3. The business office may be located at a separate area of the counter; counter space should allow for some privacy of the business office staff. This area also provides a space for patients to pay bills and schedule appointments. Conference rooms may be available for private conversations with patients.

CHAPTER 18

Basic Chairside Instruments and Tray Systems

Multiple Choice

1. a	2. b	3. d	4. c	5. b	6. c	7. d
8. c	9. d	10. c	11. b	12. c	13. b	14. b
15. c	16. c	17. a	18. b	19. c	20. b	21. c
22. c	23. b	24. b	25. c	26. b	27. c	28. c
29. d	30. b	31. a	32. c	33. d	34. a	35. c
36. b	37. b	38. d	39. b	40. d	41. c	42. c
43. c	44. a	45. b	46. c	47. d	48. b	49. c
50. b	51. c					

Matching

Match the instrument with its use.

1. e	2. a	3. d	4. c	5. b

Match each noncutting instrument with its respective use.

6. b	7. e	8. a	9. c	10. d

Match each part of the bur with its respective description.

11. b	12. c	13. a

Identify each bur name with its respective function.

14. c	15. d	16. a	17. e	18. b

Critical Thinking

1. Check for corrosion, stains, broken tips, and sharpness. After sterilization, instruments should be dried completely before being stored.

2. Corrosion and staining could occur. When the sterilization bags and the instruments within are not completely dry, they will provide a source of bacterial contamination and should be re-sterilized.

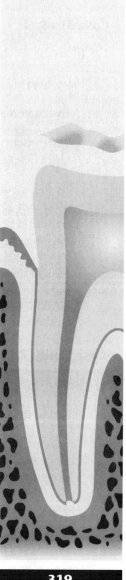

3. Burs are used for cavity preparations, finishing and polishing restorations, surgical procedures, and dental appliance adjustments.

4. Laboratory burs are used to adjust acrylic materials, such as partials, dentures, and custom trays. They are also used on plaster, stone, and metal materials. These burs are sometimes referred to as vulcanite or acrylic burs.

5. Sandpaper discs: Used to finish and polish all types of restorations and appliances. They come in a wide variety of sizes, grits, and abrasive materials, including garnet, sand, emery, and cuttlefish.

   Diamond discs: Diamond particles or chips are bonded to both sides of steel discs. Used for rapid cutting.

   Stones: Similar to discs, they are available in many sizes, shapes, and grits. Used for cutting, polishing, and finishing amalgam, gold, composite, and porcelain restorations. In the laboratory, stones are used to adjust and polish appliances and custom trays. These abrasive materials include silicon carbide, garnet, and aluminum oxide. Stones can be mounted or unmounted.

   Rubber wheels and/or points: Rubber material is impregnated with an abrasive agent. These are available mounted and unmounted, and in various grits. Used for finishing and polishing, the points are especially adaptable when defining anatomy in the restoration.

Case Study 1

1. Instruments should be cleaned as soon as possible after use.

2. Place instruments in an ultrasonic bath or other instrument washer for (manufacturer's) designated time.

   Instruments should be covered with ultrasonic solution and spread out as much as possible.

   Instrument cassettes reduce the possibility of damage to the instrument and provide more organization and efficiency. Cassettes also reduce the risk of injury to the assistant during the cleaning process.

3. Hinged instruments should always be cleaned and sterilized in the open position, as this practice prevents debris from gathering in the hinges and keeps the instruments functioning smoothly. Follow the manufacturer's directions; lubricating hinged instruments after cleaning but before sterilizing will increase instrument longevity.

4. When instruments are removed from the ultrasonic bath, they should be rinsed thoroughly under running water and then dried before being prepared for sterilization. After sterilization, instruments should be dried completely before being stored. Careful, complete evaluation and examination of all instruments should occur after sterilization and before storing.

Case Study 2

1. Round bur is used first to open the cavity and remove carious tooth structure. Bur range: 1/4, 1/2, 1, 2, 3, 4.

2. Inverted cone bur is used to remove caries and make undercuts in the preparation. Bur range: 33 1/2, 34, 35, 36. "L" indicates long.

3. Plain fissure straight bur is used to form the cavity walls of the preparation. Bur range: 56, 57, 58. The cross-cut bur comprises the taper blade plus a cross-cut.

4. Tapered fissure straight bur is used to form divergent walls of the cavity preparation. Bur range: 169–172 and 169L–171L

Case Study 3

1. Binangle chisel has two angles in the shanks of the instrument. It is used in Class II cavity preparations (MO, DO). (See Figure 18-8B in textbook.)

2. Enamel hatchet has an angle in the shank of the hatchet and the blade is fat. The hatchet is used in a downward motion to refne the cavity walls and to obtain retention in the cavity preparation. (See Figure 18-10B in textbook.)

3. Gingival (mesial) marginal trimmers (GMTs) are similar to the hatchet but the blade on GMTs is curved, not fat like the hatchet. The cutting edge is at an angle, not straight across like the hatchet. This is a double-ended instrument, and one end curves toward the mesial. These trimmers are used to bevel the mesial gingival margin wall of the cavity preparation. (See Figure 18-12D in textbook.)

4. Like the mesial marginal trimmer, the distal marginal trimmer is used to bevel the distal gingival margin wall of the cavity preparation. (See Figure 18-12B in textbook.)

Instrument Transfer and Maintaining the Operating Field

True or False

1. a   2. b   3. a   4. a   5. a   6. b   7. a

8. b   9. b   10. a

Multiple Choice

1. d   2. d   3. b   4. c   5. c   6. d   7. b

8. d   9. a   10. d

Matching

Match the term with the best description.

1. d   2. a   3. b   4. c

Match each grasp type with its best definition.

5. b   6. c   7. d   8. a

Match each transfer step with its description.

9. b   10. c   11. a

Critical Thinking

1.   a. Used to isolate an area, rest the HVE on, place materials with, or serve as something for the patient to bite on.

     b. Placed using cotton pliers or directly placed (with fingers) in the mouth by the dentist or the dental assistant.

     c. Placed on the buccal side (cheek side) of the teeth, both maxillary and mandibular arches; in the vestibule area (the pocket formed by the soft tissues of the cheeks and the gingiva, sometimes referred to as the mucobuccal fold); on the lingual side of the mandible (the tongue is gently retracted and the cotton roll is placed between the lingual surfaces of the teeth and the base of the tongue).

     d. Use either cotton pliers or directly remove from the mouth. When cotton rolls are moist, they remove easily. When dry, they should be moistened with water before removal.

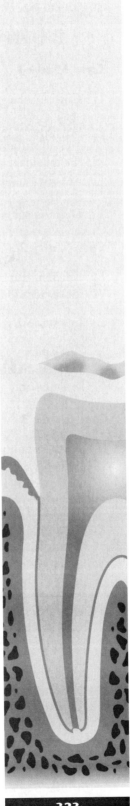

2. a. The assistant picks up the mirror in the right hand and the explorer in the left hand to transfer to a right-handed operator. The operator signals readiness by placing his or her hands in position. The assistant then simultaneously places both instruments in the operator's hands.

    b. Two-handed transfer/action, which occurs simultaneously, even though at this point there is no added exchange.

3. a. The operator may have to back away from the patient's mouth to receive certain instruments.

    b. Size and weight of certain instruments may require transfer modification.

Case Study 1

1. Cotton rolls, dry angles, and a dental dam.

2. Cotton rolls are flexible and easily placed, and can be placed in both buccal and lingual locations. Dry angles (absorbent wafers) are triangular absorbent pads that protect the cheek. They are placed directly on the maxillary and mandibular buccal mucosa, and provide a surface for cheek retraction. Both methods will absorb saliva and help to control moisture in these areas. A dental dam allows better visualization of the area the dentist is working on and controls moisture by ensuring the tooth surface remains dry when bonding agents, etchants, and restorative materials are used.

Case Study 2

1. Efficient transfer enables the operator to keep his or her eyes focused on the oral cavity and requires little movement of the operator's hands.

2. In a smooth transfer, the assistant is able to transfer and anticipate the operator's needs.

3. The operator's view remains on the oral cavity. Stress and fatigue for the operator and the assistant are reduced. Safety and comfort are maintained for the patient. Production is increased in less time and with less motion.

Case Study 3

1. The assistant passes and receives instruments with the left hand when working with a right-handed dentist and with the right hand when assisting a left-handed operator. Using one hand for instrument transfer frees the other hand for evacuation and retraction.

    Efficient instrument transfer allows the operator to keep his or her eyes focused on the oral cavity and requires little movement of the operator's hand. In sit-down, four-handed dentistry, one of the basic functions is the instrument transfer. The skill to pass and receive instruments to the operator allows efficiency and safety. When successful, the operator and assistant work as one.

2. A sequence for one-handed instrument transfer includes the following movements: approach, retrieval, and delivery. The assistant picks up the next instrument to be transferred with one hand and with the same hand receives the instrument the operator is finished using. Immediately after receiving the used instrument, the dental assistant rotates the new instrument into the operator's hand.

    The two-handed transfer is the most common. It saves time and allows the assistant to use the evacuator or the air-water syringe at the same time. The assistant uses both hands for the exchange—one to receive the used instrument from the operator and the other hand to pass the next instrument to the operator. This transfer is used most commonly for surgical forceps or when both hands are free, as well as for dental handpieces and the air-water syringe.

3. The operator will usually signal a transfer upon tilting the instrument away from the patient while still maintaining the fulcrum. The assistant removes the used instrument from the operator's hand and places the new instrument in it.

Anesthesia and Sedation

Multiple Choice

1. c	2. d	3. a	4. a	5. b	6. c	7. d
8. b	9. c	10. c	11. b	12. b	13. d	14. d
15. d	16. d	17. d	18. c	19. c	20. b	21. d
22. d	23. d	24. d	25. a	26. b	27. b	28. a
29. b	30. b	31. b				

Matching

Match the injection site with the teeth most affected.

1. d	2. c	3. a	4. b

Match the part with its function.

5. d	6. e	7. b	8. c	9. a

Critical Thinking

1. One prescribed way is as a sedative hypnotic, and the other is as an anti-anxiety drug. A sedative hypnotic will keep the patient calm and drowsy, and an anti-anxiety drug will keep the patient very calm and relaxed.

2. a. Immediately squeeze the area of the needlestick or puncture to make it bleed.

   b. Go to a sink and wash the wound area with antimicrobial soap.

   c. Notify the dentist and find out which patient the instrument was used on.

   d. Review the patient's chart and medical history.

   e. Follow Occupational Safety and Health Administration (OSHA) protocol for occupational exposure to bloodborne pathogens.

3. a. The type of injection given.

   b. Type of topical and local anesthetic administered.

   c. If the anesthetic contains a vasoconstrictor.

   d. Percentage of solution.

   e. Number of carpules used.

   f. Any patient reactions.

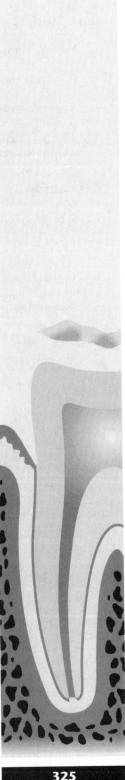

Case Study 1

1. Benzodiazepine is a commonly prescribed drug to reduce anxiety. In this instance, the drug will be used as an anti-anxiety drug rather than a sedative hypnotic.

2. Very calm and relaxed.

3. It should be taken the night before the appointment. Relieves stress for the patient and helps her to get a good night's rest.

Case Study 2

1. For the right side.

2. Posterior superior alveolar nerve block.

3. Apex of the second molar toward the distobuccal root.

4. The maxillary second and third molars, distobuccal and palatal roots of the first molar. Buccal tissues adjacent to these teeth.

Case Study 3

1. Syringe, needles, cartridge.

2. Tighten if loose when preparing and again before syringe transfer.

3. Short, 1 inch; long, 1-5/8".

4. Red—lidocaine 2% with epinephrine, 1:100,000; brown—mepivacaine 2% with levonordefrin, 1:20,000.

Introduction to Dental Radiography and Equipment

Multiple Choice

1. b	2. c	3. a	4. d	5. a	6. d	7. d
8. b	9. b	10. d	11. c	12. a	13. b	14. a
15. c	16. d	17. b	18. a	19. b	20. b	21. b
22. b	23. c	24. c	25. b	26. d	27. c	28. b
29. a	30. c					

Matching

Match each type of radiation with the best definition.

1. c   2. b   3. d   4. a

Match each x-ray tube component with its respective function.

5. d   6. a   7. b   8. e   9. c

Match each film size with its respective use.

10. e   11. d   12. b   13. a   14. c

Critical Thinking

1. Parts: outer package and black paper, dental film, black paper, lead foil backing, outer package. (See also Figure 21-15 in text to identify components.)

2. D-speed, called Ultraspeed. E-speed film, called Ektaspeed, requires approximately 40% less exposure time than Ultraspeed. F-speed film, called InSight, requires 60% less exposure time than D-speed film and 20% less exposure time than E-speed film. InSight is the highest-speed dental film, and patient radiation exposure is the lowest.

3. Long round PID: 50% reduction is noted in the thyroid area when using a lead apron with a thyroid collar. The long round PID without a lead apron results in an exposure of 0.5 mrad; with a lead apron, exposure is approximately 0.01 mrad. Rectangular PID reduces radiation exposure by approximately 60%.

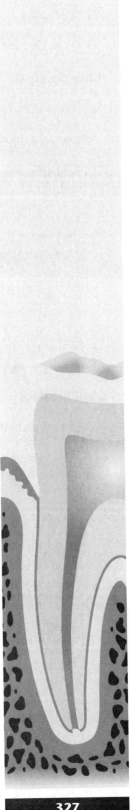

Case Study 1

1. No. 2.

2. No. 1.

3. No. 3.

4. A No. 4. Occlusal film. See Table 21.3, or Fig. 21.14

   Note: Occlusal films are used: No. 4 for adults and No. 2 for children

Case Study 2

1. The control panel comprises the circuit board and controls that allow the operator to adjust settings for each patient. The settings in this case (for Sue, an adult) would be maxillary, first molar—the area of the oral cavity requiring diagnostic x-ray exposure.

2. Milliamperage (mA) is the measurement unit for electrical current. The higher the mA, the greater the amount of radiation.

3. Kilovolts (kV) determine the quality or penetrating power of the central beam. The higher the kilovolts, the greater the penetration of the x-rays and the less exposure time required. Therefore, the patient is exposed to less radiation at higher kilovolt levels compared to lower ones.

4. The timer controls the total time that energy flows from the x-ray tube. It is a rotating dial with which the dental assistant selects the number of fractions of a second or impulses that are needed to produce the x-ray. (In Sue's case, a predetermined setting is posted near the control panel.)

5. Milliamperage (mA) determines the amount of radiation exposure the patient receives. Once set, most offices do not change the kVp and mA, except for child and adult variations.

Case Study 3

1. "As low as reasonably achievable," a concept that all dental personnel use for protection against radiation.

2. The embryo is very sensitive to radiation. Radiation of an embryo may cause death, congenital disorders, or growth retardation. Every precaution is taken if pregnancy is suspected. All pregnant patients should receive protection with lead aprons with thyroid collars during radiation exposure.

3. Tissues that are radiosensitive in the dental region are the lens of the eye and the thyroid gland.

4. Maximum permissible dose (MPD) is the maximum dose of radiation that, in light of present knowledge, would not be expected to produce any significant health effects in the course of a lifetime.

5. Natural and artificial.

6. The latent period occurs between direct exposure and development of biological effects (symptoms). "Long-term effect" means that the effects of radiation are cumulative. The health effects of exposure increase every time the individual is exposed to radiation.

CHAPTER 22

Production and Evaluation of Dental Radiographs

Multiple Choice

1. a	2. c	3. a	4. b	5. a	6. a	7. a
8. b	9. a	10. a	11. b	12. d	13. b	14. d
15. d	16. d	17. a	18. c	19. a	20. b	

Matching

Match the area with the vertical angulation.

1. c   2. a   3. d   4. b

Labeling

1–3. See Figure 22–4 in textbook.

4.   See Figure 22–28 in textbook.

5.   See Figure 22–27 in textbook.

Critical Thinking

1. Bite-wing x-rays are taken at intervals of 6 to 12 months for caries detection. They also assist in the evaluation and/or detection of restorations, calculus, alveolar crestal bone, tooth eruption, occlusal relationships, and certain pulpal pathology.

2. In labial mounting, the raised dot is toward the operator as if the operator were facing the patient. In lingual mounting, the depressed dot (concave side) is toward the operator as if the operator is viewing the films from the inside out (from a position inside the oral cavity looking outward).

3. Ensure that the film is evenly placed in the holder. Allow no more than one-eighth inch to extend beyond the edge of the occlusal plane. Once the film and film holder are in the patient's mouth, recheck that the dot on the film is toward the occlusal/incisal surface.

Case Study 1

1. Crowns, interproximal spaces, and crest area of the alveolar bone of both the maxillary and mandibular teeth.

2. Interproximal radiographs.

3. Posterior perspective.

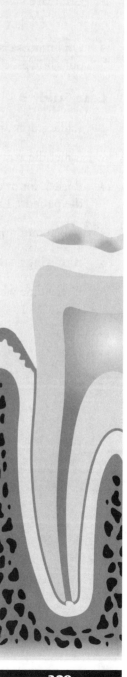

4. Premolar and molar areas, and is most often placed in a horizontal position.

5. Caries, faulty restorations, calculus, and the crestal area of the alveolar bone.

6. Horizontal positioning—angulations are needed on the premolars and molars to open the contacts. Film size and number depend on the patient's mouth. Vertical positioning—usually requested by the periodontist as well as the general dentist. This positioning will show more of the root area. Can be used in both anterior and posterior areas.

Case Study 2

1. Detects caries, abscesses, cysts, anodontia, fractures, and eruption stages and growth patterns.

2. No.

3. Compared to adults, radiation exposure time for children is reduced, and the number of radiographs must be reduced to a minimum.

4. Oral mucosa is sensitive to the slightest pressure. Check carefully for loose or erupting teeth; any parulis, pulp polyps, cold sores, and canker sores; or any deviation from the normal.

Case Study 3

1. Radiographs, lighted viewbox, x-ray mount (using full-mouth, 18 x-ray mount), and clean dry surface.

2. Label the x-ray mount with the patient's name and the date of the exposure, in pencil.

3. Raised dot or convex side is toward the operator. The operator views the film as if she or he were facing the patient. This is called labial mounting.

4. Labial mounting.

5. Bite-wings, anterior periapicals, and posterior periapicals.

6. Determine whether all x-rays are mounted similarly to the position of the teeth in the mouth.

CHAPTER 23

Extraoral and Digital Radiography

Multiple Choice

1. d	2. d	3. b	4. c	5. d	6. a	7. d
8. d	9. a	10. d	11. b	12. c	13. d	14. a
15. d	16. a	17. c	18. d	19. b	20. c	

Matching

Match each dental x-ray unit with appropriate patient positioning.

1. c   2. b   3. a

Match each component of the panoramic unit with its function.

4. c   5. d   6. b   7. a

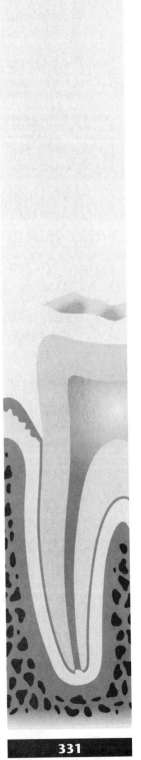

Labeling

See Figure 23-24 in the textbook.

See Figure 23-22 in the textbook.

Critical Thinking

1. Lead aprons with thyroid collars are not to be used when performing a panoramic exposure. The collar on most people is too large and closes around the chin.

2. When sensors are used, there is less exposure to radiation for the patient, and the dentist has quick results with the image appearing on the monitor almost immediately after exposure to x-rays. Initial expense of the equipment is a disadvantage and the sensors are usually thicker than the x-ray film.

3. Three-dimensional imaging allows the dental specialist to see more detail in the radiograph and allows better visualization of the relationships between the anatomical structures. The procedures can often be completed right in the dental office. The images can be taken with the patient either standing or sitting. The software can problem solve anatomical problems to aid in diagnosing and treatment planning.

Case Study 1

1. a. Under safety light conditions, load the cassette in the darkroom.

    b. Place panoramic film between the two cassette-intensifying screens.

    c. The cassette must be firmly closed to prevent light leakage.

    d. After labeling, place the cassette into machine's cassette holder.

    e. Prepare the bite-block and place barrier on it.

    f. Adjust the machine to the patient's approximate height, and set the kV and mA according to manufacturer's guidelines.

2. Patient name, date, and dentist name.

3. The bite-block will have a protective barrier.

4. a. Explain the procedure to the patient and ask if he or she has any questions.

    b. Ask patient to remove eyeglasses, earrings, tongue bars, facial piercing materials, hair pins/clips, necklaces, hearing aids, and partial/full dentures.

    c. Place and secure lead apron on the patient (lead apron without collar) (apron has two parts—one for the front and connecting back).

    d. Guide patient into position whether sitting or standing. Ask the patient to stand/sit as straight as possible, keeping vertebral column perfectly straight.

    e. Raise the machine to an appropriate level so that the patient can easily bite on the bite-block.

    f. Have the patient move forward until upper and lower teeth are secured in the groove on the bite-block. If the patient is edentulous, the alveolar ridges should be positioned over the grooves of the bite-block.

    g. Cotton rolls can assist in proper positioning.

    h. Turn the light on and adjust patient accordingly.

    i. Have midsagittal plane/Frankfort plane positioned.

    j. Instruct patient to remain still during exposure.

5. The midsagittal plane divides the face into right to left halves. The Frankfort plane is an imaginary line from the middle of the ear to just below the eye socket across the bridge of the nose.

Case Study 2

1. a. Anatomic landmarks assist in identification for mounting x-rays and communicating with the dentist and the patient.

    b. Radiopaque structures are dense and do not allow x-rays to pass through them. The structures show up in light gray to white shades on the x-ray depending on density.

    c. Radiolucent structures show up on x-rays in shades of dark gray to black. The structure is not dense, and x-rays penetrate in varying degrees.

2. a. Radiopaque area on the crown of teeth.

   b. Area just inferior to enamel; less radiopaque than enamel.

   c. Radiopaque, like dentin; thin covering on the root(s).

   d. Radiolucent area surrounded by dentin. The pulp horns can be seen on the x-ray; projections typically correspond with cusps of the tooth.

   e. Radiolucent areas in the root, which extend from pulp chamber to the apex of tooth.

   f. Radiolucent area that surrounds the root(s) of tooth.

   g. Radiopaque line of cortical bone that surrounds the root(s) of tooth and periodontal ligament.

   h. Dense compact bone that forms tooth socket.

   i. Alveolar bone found between tooth roots; radiopaque on x-ray.

   j. Alveolar bone found between adjacent teeth; shows radiopaque.

3. Possible answers are:

   (s) symphysis, (ac) alveolar crest, (mc) mandibular canal, (mrp) mandibular retromandibular pad, (cor) coronoid, (msn) medial sigmoid notch, (c) condyle, (eor) external oblique ridge, (mf) mental foramen, (bom) border of mandible.

4. Possible answers are:

   (mt) maxillary tuberosity, (eam) external auditory meatus, (gf) glenoid fossa, (ms) maxillary sinus, (o) orbit, (nf) nasal fossa, (ns) nasal septum, (nc) nasa conchae, (hp) hard palate, (i) Incisive foramen, (m) mastoid process, (zp) zygomatic process

Case Study 3

1. a. Turn on the computer, check to see that the computer screen has been activated, and select the type of radiograph to be exposed.

   b. Enter the patient's identification information and the date.

   c. Select the sensor that has been either disinfected or sterilized and placed.

   d. Place appropriate barrier over the sensor.

   e. Place the sensor into the appropriate x-ray film holder.

   f. Prepare the x-ray machine and adjust the settings.

2. a. Seat the patient so that the midsagittal plane is perpendicular to the floor.

   b. Adjust the chair to a comfortable level.

   c. Adjust the headrest to position the patient's head so that the occlusal plane is parallel to the floor.

   d. Place lead apron with the thyroid collar on the patient.

   e. Request that the patient remove eyeglasses and any objects from the mouth that might interfere with the procedure.

   f. Quickly inspect the oral cavity for anything that may require altering placement of the sensor.

3. a. Place the sensor in the patient's mouth and carefully move into position for exposure.

    b. Align the x-ray cone and PID to direct the central rays.

    c. Using the keyboard or mouse, activate the sensor to expose.

    d. Press the exposure button to expose the sensor.

    e. Wait until the image appears on the monitor to evaluate the image and determine whether a retake is necessary.

Endodontics

Multiple Choice

1. d	2. c	3. d	4. b	5. c	6. d	7. a
8. b	9. d	10. b	11. c	12. c	13. b	14. d
15. c	16. d	17. d	18. d	19. c	20. b	21. b
22. a	23. b	24. a	25. b	26. a	27. b	28. a
29. b	30. b	31. b	32. d	33. b	34. d	35. c

Matching

Match instrument image to the name of the instrument.

1. b   2. c   3. a

Critical Thinking

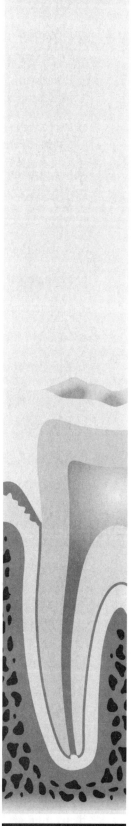

1. The general dentist sends written instructions and radiographs. The endodontist also often communicates with the referring dentist concerning the patient's treatment and prognosis. The patient may return to the general dentist for the final restoration.

2. The endodontic spoon excavator removes deep caries, pulp tissue, and temporary cement.

   The endodontic explorer, specifically designed for endodontics, helps locate canal orifices (openings).

   Endodontic spreaders have pointed ends to laterally condense materials when obturating (sealing/filling) the canal.

   Endodontic pluggers have ends, also known as condensers, to condense the filling material to provide space for additional gutta percha cones.

   The Glick #1 is used to remove excess gutta percha from the coronal portion of the canal and to condense the remaining gutta percha in the canal opening.

3. Extraoral examination: Evaluate facial asymmetry, swelling, redness, and external fistulas, and any symptoms experienced by patient.

   Intraoral examination: Look for any abnormalities or signs of inflammation, caries, discoloration, and fractures.

   Other tests include palpation, pressure applied to mucosal tissue near apex of root of suspicious tooth, percussion, tapping on the occlusal or incisal surface of the tooth, mobility (teeth that move 2 to 3 mm are not appropriate for root canal therapy), cold/hot tests for vitality, electrical pulp testing, transillumination to check for fractures, and caries removal to determine pulp condition.

Case Study 1

1. Facial asymmetry, swelling, redness, and external fistulas, and any symptoms reported by Ed.

2. a. Palpation of the soft tissues, the mucosal tissue near the apex of root of suspicious tooth. One or more additional teeth are also palpated for comparison.

   b. Percussion, by tapping, on the occlusal, or incisal surface. The handle of the mouth mirror is often used to tap the tooth or teeth.

   c. Mobility is determined by the condition and involvement of the supporting structures of the tooth or teeth. Teeth that move 2 to 3 mm are inappropriate for root canal therapy.

3. Other tests include cold test, heat test, electric pulp testing/vitality, transillumination test, selective anesthesia, and caries removal.

4. a. Administer the anesthetic.

   b. Isolate the area.

   c. Gain access to the pulp.

   d. Locate the canals.

   e. Remove the pulpal tissues.

   f. Enlarge and smooth the root canal.

   g. Irrigate the root canal.

   h. Place temporary filling.

   i. Obturate (seal) the root canal.

   j. Refer the patient to a general dentist for final restoration.

Case Study 2

1. Intracanal instruments have precise diameters and lengths that are consistent from manufacturer to manufacturer. They range in size from 08 to 140, and in length from 21 to 25 mm. Next, these instruments are flexible and able to maintain sharp cutting edges. Wire is twisted and tapered into instruments called files and reamers.

2. a. Barbed broaches are made of fine metal wire with tiny, sharp projections or barbs along the instrument shaft. Used to remove soft tissue from the pulp canal (extirpate). The dentist selects a broach that is large enough to remove pulpal tissue but small enough so that it will not bind in the canal.

   b. Files are used to enlarge and smooth the canal. They are long, tapered, and twisted, and move up and down inside the canal. Standard files are known as K-type files.

   c. Reamers are used with a "reaming" or twisting motion. They have long, twisted shanks like the files, but their blades are spaced much farther apart. Reamers are not used as frequently as files.

3. These instruments attach to a slow-speed handpiece. They have a notched end that attaches to the handpiece and are specifically designed for use in endodontic procedures. Known as rotary or engine instruments, these instruments include broaches, files, and reamers.

4. Endodontic spoon excavator—Removes deep caries, pulp tissue, and temporary cement. It has a very long shank, which allows the instrument to reach into the coronal portion of the tooth.

   Endodontic explorer—Designed to help locate canal orifices. Double-ended instrument with long, tapered ends with sharp points. Stiff-ended explorer designed specifically for endodontic procedures.

   Endodontic spreaders—Used to laterally condense materials when obturating (sealing/filling) the canal. Spreaders adapt gutta percha into the canal, and are pointed on the ends.

   Pluggers—Used to condense the filling material to provide space for additional gutta percha cones. Pluggers are flat on the ends.

   Glick #1 instrument—Used to remove excess gutta percha from the coronal portion of the canal and to condense the remaining gutta percha in the canal opening.

5. Absorbent paper points, gutta percha, irrigation solutions, sealers/cements, and root canal disinfectant.

Case Study 3

1. Narrow or curved canals were not treated during first treatment; complicated canal anatomy, such as supplemental canals, went undetected; and restoration was not placed soon enough after treatment.

2. The endodontist would reopen the tooth to gain access to the root canal. This may be difficult to accomplish when the tooth has a crown, post, and core material, all of which must be removed to permit access.

3. After removing restorative materials, canals will be cleaned and carefully examined. The problem could be supplemental canals and/or unusual anatomy. After cleaning the canals, the canal will be filled and sealed and a temporary filling will be placed. The patient then returns to the general dentist.

4. Apicoectomy.

Oral and Maxillofacial Surgery

True or False

1. a　　2. a　　3. b　　4. b　　5. a　　6. a　　7. b

8. b　　9. b　　10. a

Multiple Choice

1. d　　2. b　　3. b　　4. c　　5. d　　6. d　　7. b

8. c　　9. c　　10. d　　11. d　　12. c　　13. c　　14. d

15. b　　16. b　　17. b　　18. b　　19. a　　20. b　　21. b

22. c　　23. d　　24. a　　25. d　　26. d　　27. d　　28. c

29. c　　30. b　　31. a　　32. d　　33. a　　34. d　　35. a

Matching

Match the elevator type with its use.

1. c　　2. d　　3. a　　4. b

Match the oral surgery instrument with the photo of the instrument.

1. e　　2. d　　3. a　　4. b　　5. c

Critical Thinking

1. The healing process should not be disturbed when removing the sutures. The suture is removed with the least amount of trauma to the tissues. All sutures are removed from the suture site. The knot is not cut.

2. The surgical scrub was commonly referred to as the "5-minute scrub," but an important study indicated that scrub times of 3 to 4 minutes are just as effective. Follow the scrub product manufacturer's instructions and OSHA guidelines. Do not use a brush so stiff that it creates tiny skin abrasions. Typically, the surgical scrub includes the hands and forearms up to the elbows.

3. Surgical scalpels are surgical knives used to incise or excise soft tissue precisely with the least amount of trauma. Blade 15 is for surgical procedures, and blades #11 and #12 are used to incise and drain.

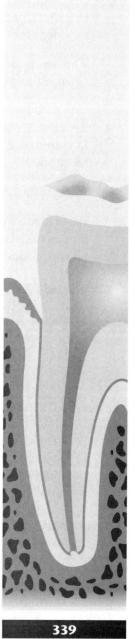

Case Study 1

1. Instructions are provided routinely after oral surgery. Postoperative home care instructions are provided by the dental assistant at the direction of the surgeon. The instructions are given verbally to the patient and the patient's escort. In addition, a written copy of the instructions with the office phone number is given to the patient, along with necessary prescriptions.

2. Discomfort reaches a peak when the anesthetic wears off and sensation returns. Swelling is normal following a surgical procedure. The swelling will continue up to 24 hours after surgery and can persist for 4 to 5 days. Facial discoloration may appear but will disappear in a day or so. Bleeding or oozing may occur for the first 12 to 24 hours after surgery. The surgeon will place a sterile gauze in your mouth to bite on immediately following surgery. Remove the gauze when the oozing has stopped. Difficulty opening the mouth, a sore throat, and earaches are not uncommon, especially if third molars were removed.

3. Begin taking pain medication before the discomfort begins and the anesthetic wears off. The surgeon will prescribe a stronger medication for pain control, if necessary. Take medications as directed to avoid nausea and vomiting. Use ice pack 20 minutes on and 20 minutes off. Apply the pack to the face over the extraction site. Continue this cycle intermittently throughout the first 12 to 24 hours. If the swelling has not subsided after 48 hours, use moist heat.

   The best means to control bleeding is pressure. Place folded gauze over the surgical site and bite down. Change the sterile gauze pads as needed. If the bleeding persists, insert a wet tea bag over the surgical site and bite down for about 20 minutes.

4. Avoid strenuous physical activity for 48 hours. Do not suck through a straw, and avoid spitting. Do not smoke or chew gum. Do not drive, drink alcohol, or operate machinery while taking pain medication.

5. Contact the office. The dentist's name and phone number should be included in the written instructions.

6. Postoperative care instructions are different for implants. Examples of differences include (a) only clear liquids are taken the first 2 days after surgery; (b) more dietary instructions are given; and (c) use of extra pillows to elevate the head the first 2 nights after surgery.

Case Study 2

1. Alveolitis.

2. Extreme pain, foul breath and taste, exposed bone, and an empty socket.

3. Loss of blood clot leaves a dry socket, which is painful. Between the third and the fifth day after surgery symptoms usually develop. The blood clot either does not form or it forms and is lost. Mandibular third molars seem to be the most frequent sites for dry socket.

4. An anesthetic may be administered. Sutures are removed, and the surgeon may gently curettage the area of the socket to stimulate the formation of a new blood clot. The socket is gently irrigated with warm saline solution, and the alveolus is gently packed with a medicated dressing. The patient is scheduled to return in 1 to 2 days to repeat the process.

Case Study 3

1. Yes.

2. Oral surgeon's office.

3. Impacted third molar extractions include depth, position, or angulation of the tooth in the bone. Teeth may be impacted in soft tissue or in the bone. When impacted in bone, dental handpieces and surgical burs are required to gain access.

4. The dental assistant prepares and transfers the anesthetic and/or assists with the IV, transfers instruments such as the periosteal elevator, suctions and retracts tissue, transfers handpiece and burs, transfers forceps, transfers gauze, assists with suturing, prepares the irrigating syringe, and provides postoperative care instructions.

Oral Pathology

Multiple Choice

1. d	2. d	3. b	4. c	5. b	6. d	7. d
8. a	9. b	10. d	11. d	12. d	13. d	14. b
15. b	16. d	17. d	18. d	19. c	20. b	21. b
22. b	23. c	24. a	25. c	26. c	27. b	28. d
29. a	30. c	31. b	32. b	33. c	34. b	35. a
36. b	37. a	38. b	39. b	40. b		

Matching

Match the term with definition.

1. c   2. d   3. b   4. a

Critical Thinking

1. Hematomas are lesions caused by bleeding from a ruptured blood vessel that appear to be raised bruised areas due to collection of localized clotted blood. Even the best clinicians may nick a blood vessel during an injection, resulting in a hematoma.

2. The assistant avoids stretching and pulling the lesion, which causes pain and significant discomfort to the patient. Pay special attention to means of eliminating cross-contamination and maintaining asepsis.

3. Tongue, cheeks, lips, uvula, and the side of the tongue. Sometimes multiple sites are pierced. Tongue swelling that can close off the airway and prevent breathing is a serious side effect of piercing.

Case Study 1

1. Biological, physical, and chemical agents.

2. Hormonal, developmental, and nutritional disturbances will present symptoms in the mouth.

3. Reactions to stress and antigenic substances, as well as neoplasms and cysts.

4. Basically, abnormal conditions. Know how to prevent disease transmission, how the identified pathological condition may interfere with the planned treatment, and what effect the condition will have on the overall health of the patient.

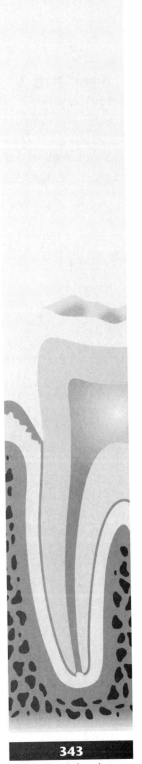

Case Study 2

1. Anything that appears to be atypical should be brought to the attention of the dentist for further investigation, without alarming the patient.

2. Any unusual oral lesions (an all-encompassing term for abnormal structures in the oral cavity) must be closely observed by the dentist. The dentist may palpate (feel with fingers) or perform a biopsy on the suspicious lesion.

3. Biopsy, the surgical removal of a small amount of the tissue from a suspicious lesion, improves accuracy in diagnosing many illnesses.

4. Cause or origins of the disease. The biopsy is normally sent to a pathologist, along with the dentist's clinical observations and results of the palpation such as size, location, color, and texture.

Case Study 3

1. Clinical assessment, genetic history, surgery, microscopic biopsy, and laboratory diagnosis. New tools are also aiding in this type of diagnosis such as the VELscope and Vizilite.

2. Visuals of the apical area, which provide data on whether areas of absorption have occurred. Also makes cysts or abscesses visible.

3. Access the location, size, shape, color, and texture of the lesion.

4. Therapeutic diagnosis, such as prescribing an antibiotic to determine whether the condition improves or is eliminated. Differential diagnosis. The conditions could be idiopathic, meaning that the disease or disorder has no known cause. The diagnosis would then be about the disease only.

Orthodontics

Multiple Choice

1. d	2. d	3. a	4. c	5. b	6. d	7. d
8. b	9. c	10. b	11. c	12. b	13. d	14. b
15. b	16. c	17. b	18. b	19. b	20. b	21. b
22. a	23. b	24. b	25. a	26. b	27. c	28. b
29. a	30. d					

Matching

Match the commonly used orthodontic instrument with its function.

1. c   2. a   3. b   4. d

Match the instrument in the photo with the proper name of the instrument.

5. c   6. d   7. a   8. b

Critical Thinking

1. a. Take study models, clean patient's teeth at various stages of treatment, take intraoral and extraoral radiographs, prefit bands before cementation, and apply sealants to teeth to be bonded.

   b. Do the tracing on cephalometric radiographs, maintain and sterilize instruments, maintain inventory and supplies, perform routine equipment maintenance, and help the dentist present the treatment plan during the consultation appointment.

2. Application of separators, placement of posterior bands, placement of anterior brackets, placement of arch wire, interval checkups, and completion appointment.

3. Glass ionomer, polycarboxylate, and zinc phosphate.

Case Study 1

1. Overbite, vertical overlap. In a normal bite, the maxillary teeth extend vertically over the incisal by one-third of the mandibular anterior teeth. An overbite exists when the overlap is more than one-third.

   Overjet, horizontal overlap. An abnormal horizontal distance between the labial surface of the mandibular anterior teeth and the lingual surface of the maxillary anterior teeth.

2. Extensive examination of the face, jaws, and teeth, looking for symmetry.

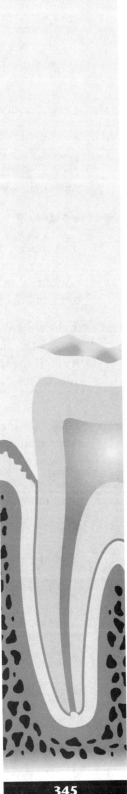

The teeth are evaluated for size, shape, color, and position.

The jaws are examined for size, shape, and relationship to one another.

The angle classification of occlusion is often used to determine whether the occlusion is the same on both sides of the mouth.

3. Panoramic view of dentition, surrounding area, impacted teeth, abscesses, supernumerary teeth, or disorders of the temporomandibular joint.

Cephalometric radiograph is taken to evaluate the growth patterns and to determine the course of treatment. It is a lateral view of the patient's head that shows the jaw and teeth. Tracings are done to determine the relationship of certain landmarks.

4. Before the consultation appointment, radiographs and study models have been collected and prepared; visual aids are also prepared.

During the consultation, the treatment, duration of treatment, involvement, and costs are explained. The patient understands his or her responsibilities in terms of what must be done to facilitate treatment progress as planned. When the patient accepts the treatment plan, consent papers are signed and financial arrangements are made; treatment can begin.

Case Study 2

1. The general dentist and the pediatric dentist provide treatment. In complex cases, the general dentist works with the orthodontist on a treatment plan for the patient. Common treatments that are considered preventive and interceptive include recognizing any deviation from the normal, and observing growth patterns and development of teeth and bones.

2. Malocclusion comprises any deviation from normal occlusion, including misalignment of a single tooth, a group of teeth, or an entire arch. It is important to maintain this space until the permanent tooth begins to erupt. If the space is not held open, the adjacent teeth will drift and begin to fill the space, making it more difficult for the permanent tooth to erupt and come in straight.

3. The space maintainer is composed of a band and a wire loop soldered together. Its function is to maintain a space for the permanent tooth to erupt after the premature loss of the primary tooth. Several varieties of space maintainers are available that can be adapted to the patient's teeth

Labeling

a. mouth mirror

b. explorer

c. cotton pliers

d. separating pliers

e. separators (elastic or metal separating materials)

f. orthodontic scaler

g. Mathieu pliers

h. high-volume evacuation (HVE) tip

i. air/water syringe

j. cotton rolls

k. dental floss or tape

Pediatric Dentistry and Dental Sealants

Multiple Choice

1. b	2. c	3. d	4. b	5. c	6. d	7. b
8. a	9. c	10. a	11. c	12. a	13. c	14. d
15. d	16. b	17. d	18. c	19. b	20. d	21. b
22. a	23. d	24. c	25. b			

Critical Thinking

1. Child management skills at chairside vary from state to state and from office to office. During treatment the dental assistant supports the dentist. The dental assistant is also an educator and motivator, providing oral health instructions and preventive care.

2. Isolation throughout the procedure is necessary. Ask the patient to keep the tongue still to prevent contamination; use dental dam; place Dri Angles on both buccal and lingual of the mandibular arch and buccal on the maxillary arch; and use Garmer clamps with cotton rolls and Dri Tips to block the Stenson's duct on the buccal mucosa. Work quickly and efficiently to keep the sealant procedure time to a minimum.

3. Is this a permanent tooth or a primary/baby tooth? Place the tooth in milk, saliva, saline, or water, and transport the patient and tooth to the dental office immediately. Caution should be taken with the avulsed tooth to place it carefully in liquid and not rinse it off.

Case Study 1

1. Caries or traumatic injuries can damage both primary and permanent teeth. Clinical assessment with radiographs is carried out to determine the status of the pulp. The duration, frequency, and location of pain are recorded. The dentist also determines whether a fistula is present and the tooth is mobile, and whether there is any swelling and/or sensitivity to sound or percussion.

2. Involves removal of tissue that is potentially infected, and focuses on the reparative ability of the pulp. Choices of treatment depend on pulp status.

3. Indirect pulp treatment (IPT) is indicated if the pulp is not yet exposed. Direct pulp capping (DPC) is indicated when the pulp has been exposed through mechanical or traumatic means, but there is a chance for a favorable response.

4. For a diagnosis of nonvital pulp, therapy may be a pulpectomy, a procedure that involves complete removal of the dental pulp.

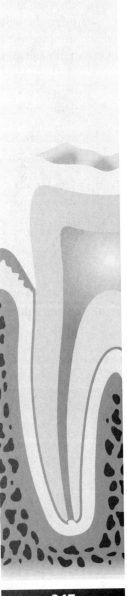

Case Study 2

1. Tell, show, and do; voice control; distraction; gentle restraints; mild sedation.

2. Subjective fears are based on feelings, attitudes, and concerns that have developed from the suggestions of others, including parents, siblings, and friends. Objective fears are based on the child's own experiences.

3. The degree of dental assistant involvement depends on the office, the situation, and the dentist. The assistant may play the dominant role in greeting the child, escorting the child to the treatment area, and preparing the child for treatment. When the dentist enters the room, the assistant transfers the attention and control to the dentist.

4. Short attention span, wide variety of interests, parallel play without bothering other children, responds to fantasy.

Case Study 3

1. The dental office provides an opportunity for abused children to be observed and for the abuse to be reported. The entire dental team needs to be aware of types of and signs of child abuse.

2. Physical abuse, sexual abuse, neglect, and emotional abuse. The injuries associated with child abuse that might be evident in the dental office include fractured teeth and jaw bones, lacerations around the labial frenum, missing teeth with no explanation, and bruises or scars on the lips. Marks on the child's arms, legs, and neck may also be noticed by the dental team. Lack of personal hygiene or appropriate clothing for the season, extensive caries, and lack of attention to the child's dental treatment needs are concerns of the dental team, and should be noted and followed up when the child's health and welfare are continually being compromised.

3. Social service agency, local police department, or child protective service. The dentist may be asked to appear in court and/or file the report.

4. The laws regarding reporting child abuse may differ from state to state, but most require the dentist to report apparent signs of abuse. The laws are designed to protect children and provide help for families.

5. The nature of the concern; description of the injury, including type, color, size, characteristics, and location; x-rays and color photographs; child's name, age, address, sex, and date of birth; parents' or caregivers' names; physician's name; and child's and caregivers' explanations of the injury.

Periodontics and Coronal Polish

Multiple Choice

1. c	2. b	3. d	4. d	5. a	6. d	7. a
8. b	9. b	10. b	11. d	12. c	13. a	14. b
15. c	16. b	17. c	18. a	19. b	20. a	21. b
22. a	23. b	24. b	25. a	26. a	27. b	28. a
29. d	30. a	31. d	32. d	33. b	34. b	35. b
36. b	37. b	38. c	39. a	40. c		

Matching

Identify the following attachments and accessories in the figure.

1. j	2. a	3. b	4. i	5. c	6. d	7. g
8. h	9. e	10. f				

Identify the periodontal instruments in the figure.

a. chisel   b. hoe   c. file

Critical Thinking

1. Use a slow, even speed, and light-to-moderate pressure. Always use a fulcrum, and start and stop the handpiece inside the patient's mouth.

2. Intrinsic stains are inside the tooth structure, whereas extrinsic stains are outside the tooth structure. Endogenous means originating from inside the tooth, and exogenous, originating from outside the tooth. Intrinsic stains can be both endogenous and exogenous. Extrinsic stains are only exogenous in origin.

3. The most common periodontal dressing materials are zinc oxide-eugenol, noneugenol, light cured, and gelatin based.

Case Study 1

1. Types of intrinsic stains: dental fluorosis, white to yellow-brown; tetracycline, light green or yellow to dark gray-brown; metallic, green to greenish blue or gray to black or bluish black.

   Types of extrinsic stains: yellow and brown, associated with poor oral hygiene; tobacco, because coal tar combustion in cigarettes penetrates pits and fissures on enamel/dentin surfaces.

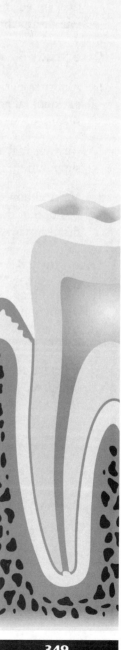

349

2. Particle shape, harness, and size.

3. The rate of abrasion is a measure of the time it takes to remove stains and deposits from a surface. The rate is based on speed of the handpiece; amount of heat, pressure, and abrasive material; and type of abrasive.

Case Study 2

1. Osseous surgery: removal of defects/deformities in the bone caused by periodontal disease and related conditions.

2. Osteoplasty: bone reshaping.

3. In additive osseous surgery, sometimes called augmentative surgery, bone or bone substitute is added as filler to the existing structure. In subtractive surgery, bone is removed or contoured.

4. A bone graft involves moving bone tissue from one area to another. Mucogingival surgery is reconstructive, aimed at covering exposed roots, increasing the width of the gingival tissue, or reducing frenum or muscle attachments. In gingival grafting, gingival tissue is taken from one site and placed on another.

Case Study 3

1. A normal periodontal sulcus measures 3 mm or less. When the depth is 3 mm or more, it is termed a periodontal pocket. Six sites per tooth—three on the facial and three on the lingual—are probed and recorded. According to the CAL scale, slight = 1 or 2 mm, moderate = 3 or 4 mm, and severe = 5 mm.

2. Answers may include: tooth mobility, furcation involvement, appearance of the gingiva, bleeding/suppuration, recession, and occlusion.

3. Vertical bone resorption is found in individual teeth on the interproximal surface showing the level and position of the alveolar bone. Horizontal bone resorption occurs when crestal bone loss on the mesial and distal surfaces of the proximal teeth is equal.

Case Study 4

1. Near-bloodless operating field so that operator's view is improved, healing time is minimized, damage to surrounding healthy tissues is reduced, and chair time is reduced.

2. Protective eyewear must be worn by the dentist, staff, and patient.

3. Sulcular debridement and laser curettage, gingivectomy, gingivoplasty, frenectomy, and implant exposure and tissue fusion, which eliminates the need for sutures.

CHAPTER 30

Fixed Prosthodontics and Gingival Retraction

Multiple Choice

1. d	2. d	3. a	4. d	5. b	6. b	7. a
8. d	9. c	10. b	11. b	12. b	13. a	14. d
15. b	16. c	17. d	18. d	19. d	20. d	

Critical Thinking

1. In mechanical retraction, the tissue can be displaced to allow access to the margin. The retraction cord is placed in the sulcus of healthy and inflamed free gingiva. The cotton cord is left in place for 10 to 15 minutes (chemical retraction cord would be left in place for 5 minutes).

   Chemical retraction, a new method, uses a topical hemostatic solution, or the retraction cord is impregnated with aluminum chloride or aluminum salt astringent. Hypertension is the main contraindication. Because the dentist will likely prefer to use a chemical retraction cord, careful review of the patient's medical history is necessary.

   As an alternative to retraction, the dentist may choose to surgically remove the tissue around the preparation via a surgical knife or electrosurgery.

2. Brushing and flossing are continued with fixed prostheses. Toothbrushes should be soft and multitufted and heads small enough to reach all areas in each quadrant. Dental floss works well under bridge work. A bridge threader can be used to run floss under the pontic and along abutment teeth. Interproximal brushes and tips are designed for removal of plaque.

   For proper care of dental implants, routine brushing and flossing are prescribed. The toothbrush should be soft and multitufted nylon. Threading systems, dental floss, interproximal brushes, water irrigators, and antimicrobial rinses are recommended.

3. Often the teeth being restored show substantial loss of tooth structure due to decay, fractures, or large deteriorated restorations. Root canal therapy may be required before the crowns and bridges are made.

   Retention options include core buildups, which are performed for vital teeth that have very little crown structure; they are made of amalgam, composite, or silver alloy/glass ionomer combinations. Retention pins provide additional retention of the core buildup. They are placed before the core buildup, and the core buildup material surrounds the pins. The number of pins depends on the amount of buildup needed or the type of restoration to follow. A post-retained core is the

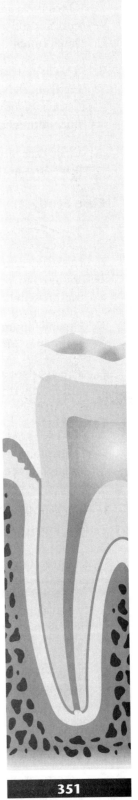

treatment of choice when the tooth is nonvital and has root canal therapy. A portion of the root canal filling is removed and a post is fitted in the canal and cemented. Posts are made of titanium, titanium alloy, gold-plated metal, and stainless steel.

Case Study 1

1. An electrosurgery unit cauterizes the tissues as it removes them.

2. Once the cauterized tissue has been removed, there is no more bleeding. The unit passes high-frequency current to a small electrode passing through the tissue. When the tip touches the tissue, the unit is activated to remove the tissue.

3. The dental assistant constantly uses a nonmetal HVE tip during electrosurgery because of the odor resulting from cauterized tissue. The evacuator reduces the odor when placed near the surgical site. After the tissue is removed, the sulcus is cleaned with a hydrogen rinse. Immediately following the procedure, the final impression is taken.

4. Electrosurgery is not used on patients who are receiving radiation therapy, have cardiac pacemakers, or have slow-healing diseases.

Case Study 2

1. The dental assistant explains the steps of the procedure to the patient and answers questions.

2. Each tray setup is arranged according to the procedure sequence, and auxiliary instruments and materials are nearby. Many types of dental materials will be utilized throughout the procedure, including bite registration materials, retraction cord, temporization materials, and final cements.

3. Expanded functions may include placing the retraction cord, placing and removing temporaries, taking preliminary impressions, and removing excess cement.

4. The assistant also coordinates patient appointments and the laboratory schedule. In some offices, the assistant may perform selected laboratory functions, such as making custom trays and pouring study models.

Case Study 3

1. Dentist and staff members must be trained to effectively use CAD/CAM restorative systems. Time devoted to practice using both the hardware and software is also necessary to become proficient. Next, such systems are expensive. The dentist and staff members should be familiar with computers, and be committed to learning the system.

2. The CEREC machine and the milling chamber.

3. Lucite-reinforced glass ceramic, fine-grained feldspathic porcelain, and a polymer.

4. Alloys are metal free, and tooth-colored restorations are fabricated in a single appointment. All types of restorations including inlays, onlays, posterior and anterior crowns, and veneers can be designed. The patient is spared unpleasant impressions and temporaries. Finally, less reduction of healthy tooth structure is required.

5. Patient is seated and anesthetized, the shade of the block ceramic material is selected, and the block is placed in the milling machine. The dentist prepares the tooth, the preparation is coated with reflective powder, and an instant optical impression is obtained by positioning the camera over the preparation. The dentist then designs the restoration using data from the CEREC software and the optical image chairside. The information is transferred to the milling machine; diamond burs work simultaneously under water coolant to mill the restoration. A try-in restoration is placed and adjustments are made as needed. Finally, the restoration is bonded and polished.

Cosmetic Dentistry and Teeth Whitening

Multiple Choice

1. b	2. c	3. b	4. c	5. b	6. a	7. c
8. d	9. d	10. c	11. d	12. c	13. c	14. b
15. b	16. a	17. b	18. b	19. d	20. c	21. d
22. b	23. d	24. a	25. d			

Matching

Match each term with its description.

1. c   2. d   3. a   4. b

Critical Thinking

1. Whitening "lightens" most teeth; some will never be the whitest or the brightest, but they will be improved. The patient's dedication to following procedures and limiting foods and habits that stain the teeth will enhance the process and whiten the teeth faster. The health of the gingiva and surrounding tissues must be protected by adhering to suggested techniques. Ingestion of lightening solutions should be kept to a minimum. The patient must realize that whitening may be an ongoing treatment, with repeated procedures necessary every few years.

2. Duties may include expanded functions such as placing and removing the rubber dam, taking detailed impressions, and creating aesthetic temporaries for the patient to wear between treatments. The assistant is available to answer the patient's questions, and provide reassurance and positive support throughout the procedure. The dental assistant may also accompany the dentist to additional training seminars, courses, and workshops, and therefore is knowledgeable about assisting with specific techniques and preparing various materials. Assistants work closely with the dentist and the patient, and may be involved in designing the right smile for a specific patient.

3. General dentistry includes many aspects of "cosmetic dentistry" and most dentists do some cosmetic dentistry. A "cosmetic dentist" needs continuing education and postgraduate-level education and additional credentialing. Many procedures are included in cosmetic/aesthetic dentistry. The cosmetic dentist performs some of the procedures; others are completed by various specialty dentists, including the orthodontist, periodontist, maxillofacial surgeon, and prosthodontist.

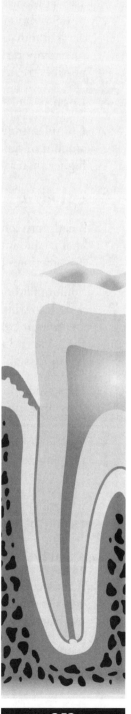

353

4. Patients are advised to get a referral, if possible, from friends and family on quality care; determine the dentist's credentials in cosmetic dentistry, and whether she or he has kept up-to-date via continuing education courses; examine before-and-after pictures of patients who have completed cosmetic dental treatments; and determine availability of appointments and possible financial arrangements.

Case Study 1

1. Extrinsic stains—yellow to brown—derive from diet deficiencies or excesses, and habits such as tobacco, tea, and coffee. Intrinsic stains derive from tetracycline, dental fluorosis, discoloration due to injury, and nonvital endodontically treated teeth. Finally, sometimes the natural shade of the teeth is yellow or gray.

2. Endodontically treated teeth sometimes turn dark due to blood, pulpal debris, and restorative materials that are used to fill the canal. Both internal and external whitening can be accomplished. One of the most common is the walking whitening technique: a thick paste of hydrogen peroxide, sodium perborate, or a combination of the two is placed in the coronal portion of the nonvital tooth. With the bleach mixture temporarily sealed in place, the patient can leave the office and return for an evaluation and another possible treatment as instructed by the dentist.

3. In-office and at-home methods.

4. Considerations include the amount of stain and its origin, the number of visits to the office versus the amount of time that the whitening trays are worn at home, the expense of the in-office whitening (which is higher than at-home whitening), and the amount of instruction and guidance the patient requires.

Case Study 2

1. Teeth turn a lighter shade when hydrogen peroxide or nonperoxide whitening material goes through the enamel and into the dentin. The whitening process is accelerated mainly by the use of low-intensity heat or sometimes by a high-intensity curing light or laser.

2. Sodium perborate (a relatively weak oxidizing agent), which is sometimes mixed with hydrogen peroxide, is used to whiten nonvital teeth. It is also an ingredient used in many household whitening agents that are safe for colors. Hydrogen peroxide solution comes in either a liquid or gel form and varies in strength from 5% to 35% in solution. Carbamide peroxide is used in a 10% to 20% solution. The latter is weaker, but more stable.

3. Depending on the office, the dental assistant may perform some or all aspects involving whitening, such as providing information and answering questions to and by patients, chairside assisting for in-office whitening treatments, providing home-care information including instructions for proper use of the whitening and care of the trays, fabricating custom whitening trays, and obtaining the informed consent form from the patient.

4. Degree of staining or discoloration, cause of the stains or discolorations, whitening technique, specific whitening solution and its strength, vital versus nonvital tooth, and whether there are restorations in the teeth to be whitened.

Case Study 3

1. This is an artistic skill that requires attention to detail and commitment by all. Everything is taken into consideration: use of natural light, principles of color and interpretation, illusion, and shape and form of teeth and gingival tissues.

2. Natural light is used when selecting the shade of teeth, as it is multidirectional and casts shadows and shows texture.

3. Color can be measured in terms of hue, chroma, and value. Hue is the name of the color, chroma is the intensity or quality of the hue, and value is the brightness of a shade.

4. Illusion is the art of making something appear to be different than it is in reality. The size and shape of teeth can be manipulated via illusion. Illusions can be created by manipulating depth, horizontal, and vertical dimensions.

5. Cultural and artistic biases affect how teeth are perceived. Included are masculine and feminine features of teeth and how the teeth are proportioned. Shaping the face of one tooth or several teeth to match each other will give the illusion that they are the same size and shape. Detail each tooth as it is and how it relates to the other teeth in the arch.

Removable Prosthodontics

True or False

1. a   2. a   3. b   4. a   5. b

Multiple Choice

1. d   2. a   3. d   4. d   5. b   6. c   7. d

8. c   9. b   10. a   11. c   12. a   13. b   14. a

15. c   16. b   17. b   18. d   19. b   20. d   21. d

22. a   23. a   24. c   25. c

Labeling

1. d   2. a   3. b   4. c

Critical Thinking

1. This is a multistep process that converts the wax try-in denture to a denture with an acrylic resin base and plastic or porcelain teeth. A dental flask is utilized for this process.

2. For an immediate denture, the baseplate and bite rims are fabricated to fit over the posterior areas only. The patient's existing anterior teeth are used for jaw relationships and measurements.

3. Examination, consultation, oral surgery, final impressions, jaw relationships, denture delivery, first follow-up (scheduled several days after the patient receives the dentures), adjustments.

Case Study 1

1. Retained teeth are treated endodontically using implants, or special prefabricated attachments and posts.

2. Retained teeth are endodontically treated with prepared posts and cores or with special prefabricated attachments.

3. Surgery is required to create a post for the implant.

4. Magnets and a "snap" design.

5. Advantages include retention and stability. Disadvantages include (a) increased cost; (b) greater time investment due to endodontic treatment, surgeries, and restorative procedures; and (c) substantial time and energy investment in maintenance of retained teeth/implant, as plaque control is necessary to prevent bone loss around the implants and/or the retained teeth to inhibit root caries.

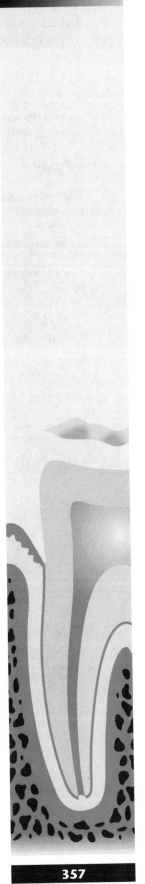

Case Study 2

1. Improves the fit of the denture and the comfort of the patient. Supporting tissues often shrink.

2. Sometimes tissues under the denture become irritated and inflamed due to an ill-fitting appliance. These tissues must be healed, which is called "tissue conditioning," before a denture reline is completed.

3. A soft reline saves the patient time, and the patient is never without the denture.

4. A laboratory reline takes more time and the patient may be without the denture for a day. A soft reline is a temporary solution, is not as durable, and will not last as long as the laboratory reline, but the patient need never be without the denture.

Case Study 3

1. The dentist examines the tissues, shapes and sizes of ridges, retromolar and tuberosity areas, frenum attachments, and undercut areas.

2. Radiographs and preliminary impressions.

3. The photographs are used as a reference to create the most natural-looking dentures possible for the patient.

4. Preparation of the diagnosis, treatment plans, and the financial estimate, all based on collected information.

Dental Cements, Bases, Liners, and Bonding Agents

Multiple Choice

1. d	2. b	3. a	4. b	5. c	6. a	7. a
8. d	9. c	10. b	11. b	12. a	13. b	14. a
15. b	16. c	17. d	18. a	19. d	20. a	21. b
22. b	23. a	24. c	25. a	26. b	27. c	28. a
29. a	30. c	31. b	32. c	33. b	34. a	35. d

Critical Thinking

1. Plastic filling instrument. Using the small condensing end of the plastic filling instrument, the base is condensed into place on the floor of the cavity preparation. Continue until sufficient base layer is placed. Cement bases are placed in the cavity preparation to protect the pulp and provide mechanical support for the restoration. These bases are placed on the floor of the cavity preparation to raise the level of the floor of the preparation to the ideal height. The type of cement used is determined by the preparation, sensitivity of the pulp, and type of restoration.

2. At the ideal level, the preparation does not involve the pulp, the preparation passes through the enamel and is in the dentin, and is large enough to retain a restoration. At the beyond-ideal level, the preparation passes through more dentin and is close to the pulp. Next is the near-exposure level, at which the cavity dentin is removed, but the pulp is not exposed. The floor of the preparation may be slightly pink due to the proximity of the pulp. Finally, at the pulp exposure level, there will be blood in the cavity preparation. Enough enamel and dentin have been removed to expose a portion of the pulp.

3. ZOP: On a cool glass slab, using a stainless steel spatula, the first increment of powder is mixed in with liquid. Wait 10 to 15 seconds before mixing in more powder. Allow heat to dissipate and continue to mix until desired consistency is achieved.

   ZOE type I: Most are mixed on a paper pad, using a stainless steel spatula; use of a glass slab will control setting time. The powder and liquid are mixed all at once. Wait 30 to 60 seconds. A uniform, smooth, creamy mix results.

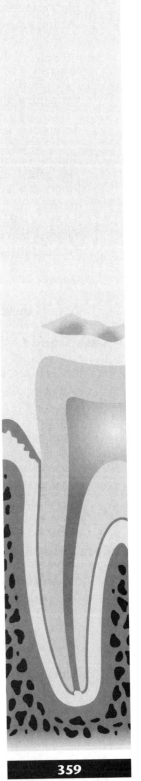

Polycarboxylate: Mix on paper pad or glass slab, using a stainless steel spatula. This material has a "cobweb" consistency. Powder and liquid are mixed; wait 30 to 60 seconds. This material is characterized by a short working time of 3 minutes.

Glass ionomer: Mix on paper pad or cool glass slab (glass slab will retard the setting action). Wait 30 to 60 seconds; follow manufacturer's directions. This material is characterized by a short working time of 2 minutes.

Calcium hydroxide: A two-paste agent, this material is mixed on a small paper pad with a metal spatula, explorer, or small ball-ended instrument. Equal portions of the pastes are mixed for about 10 to 15 seconds. Setting time varies from two to 7 minutes.

4. Luting, bonding, or cementing together: dental cements may be used as luting agents to bond inlays and bridges.

   Permanent luting cement: long-term cementing agent.

   Temporary luting cement: short-term cementing agent.

   Intermediate luting cement: material lasts 6 months to a year.

   Liner: thin layer is placed on the walls and floor of the cavity preparation. The liner protects the pulp from bacteria and irritants.

   Base: applied in putty or thick layer between the tooth and the restoration to protect the pulp from chemical irritation, temperature changes, electrical shock, and mechanical injury.

   Sedative or palliative effect: soothing effect that relieves pain but does not provide a cure.

   Varnish: thin layer applied to seal walls and floor of the cavity preparation.

Case Study 1

1. Desensitizers are used in treating or preventing hypersensitivity in teeth to heat, cold, very sugary or acidic food or drink, and contact (such as from vigorous toothbrushing).

2. Desensitizers can be used under all types of restorations and bonding agents. Etchants, which are placed before bonding agents, enhance the retention/bonding qualities between the tooth surface and dental materials.

3. The dentist used etchants and bonding agents, and thus retention between the tooth and restorative materials is likely quite good. The patient was encouraged by the dentist to wait for a short time for the sensitivity to dissipate.

Case Study 2

1. Terms pertaining to a cavity preparation include axial wall, pulpal wall or floor, gingival wall, line angle, point angles, and cavosurface margin.

2. Cutting of the tooth structure depends on the location of the decay, the extent of the decay, the amount of lost tooth structure, and the type of restorative material to be used.

3. Change burs, rinse and evacuate the oral cavity, and mix materials.

Case Study 3

1. A DIAGNOdent unit is a Class II laser that measures fluorescence levels within the tooth structure to quantify caries progression.

2. In laser detection, altered tooth structure and bacteria fluoresce when exposed to specific wavelengths of light. A clean, healthy tooth structure exhibits little or no fluorescence, while a tooth containing decay will exhibit fluorescence according to the extent of the caries.

3. Healthy teeth have low readings, and teeth containing decay will have higher readings. The dentist observes changes on a visual display as the unit explores teeth; the unit can also be programmed to provide audio signals that change as the level of caries changes.

4. Benefits of using a DIAGNOdent unit include accurate diagnosis of tooth decay; noninvasiveness; simple, fast, and painless; and early detection.

Restorative Materials, Dental Dam, Matrix, and Wedge

Multiple Choice

1. b	2. b	3. c	4. b	5. c	6. c	7. d
8. b	9. b	10. a	11. b	12. d	13. d	14. a
15. c	16. c	17. d	18. d	19. c	20. b	

Critical Thinking

1. Free the interseptal (rubber dam material in the septum space) dam with scissors. To protect the patient, slip the index or middle finger under the dam material and stretch it away from the tooth. Slant the scissors toward the occlusal surface and clip each septum with the scissors. Pulling the dam material toward the facial, the operator cuts the interseptal dam.

2. Invert or tuck the dam material. The edge of the dam that surrounds the tooth must be inverted or tucked into the sulcus of the gingiva to seal the tooth and prevent leakage. Carefully pull the dental dam material slightly apically, and the dam will often invert when it is released. When using floss to place the dam interproximally, it may be inverted. Use a T-ball burnisher, a plastic instrument, or a spoon excavator to tuck the buccal and lingual surfaces. Use the instrument with the air from the air-water syringe to dry the surface and then invert the edge of the dam. Continue until all edges of the dam are sealed.

3. Punching the arch too flat or wide results in folds or bunching and stretching on the lingual. Punching the arch too curved or narrow results in folds and stretching on the facial. The punch table should be clean and free of previously punched dam material Check for nicks in the holes of the punch table, as these will leave a tag of dam material and will tear around the punched hole.

   Hole spacing should match the space between the patient's teeth. When holes are too close together, there is not enough material to seal around each tooth. When holes are too far apart, there will be excess material and interproximal placing of the dam will be difficult.

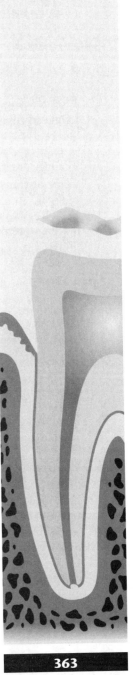

4. The purpose of clamps is to stabilize and secure the dental dam material in place.

   The selection process requires evaluation of the tooth and mesiodistal width at the CEJ of the tooth. Width of the tooth must be about the same as the width between the points of the jaws of the clamp. The faciolingual width at the CEJ of the tooth must also be estimated to ensure that the clamp fits tightly.

   The basic parts of the clamp are: (A) bow, (B) jaw, (C) forceps hole, and (D) jaw points.

5. The plastic strip matrix provides anatomic contour and proximal contact relation, prevents excess material at the gingival margin, confines the restorative material under pressure while the material is being cured, protects the restorative material from losing or gaining moisture during the setting time, and allows the polymerizing light to reach the composite restorative material. The strip matrix is thin and transparent, and can be made of nylon, acetate, celluloid, or resin. It is approximately 3 inches long and 3/8 inch wide. The plastic strip can also be used as a crown matrix form.

   The plastic strip matrix can be used with composite, glass ionomer, or compomer restorative materials on anterior teeth.

Case Study 1

1. A wedge is placed only when the preparation includes one or more proximal surfaces.

2. Pros of wedge placement are that it holds the band securely in place and prevents excess filling material from escaping between the tooth and the matrix. Cons are that excess material escapes below the matrix and that the wedge can damage the gingival tissues if left in place.

3. Wedges are available in various sizes, and colors range from transparent to natural to colored (not natural). Clear or transparent wedges are used with light-curing cement.

4. Wedges are usually placed from the lingual on posterior teeth. Cotton pliers or a hemostat are used to place and remove wedges. The smallest of the three sides is placed toward the gingiva. The wedge should fill the space and fit snugly.

Case Study 2

1. Quickdam.

2. Examine the patient's dentition and determine whether it is mixed, which primary teeth are missing (if any), and which teeth are partially erupted. Holes are punched in accordance with these conditions. Generally, the holes are punched close together. No holes are punched where teeth are missing or just barely erupted. In some cases, holes are punched only for the teeth that are directly involved.

3. The quickdam has its own template to mark each tooth. Hole sizes are the same for the quickdam and full dam.

4. After the holes have been punched, the dam frame is folded and inserted into the patient's mouth; the dam is then fitted around the teeth to be isolated.

5. The quickdam does not require the use of a clamp, but a clamp may be used at the operator's discretion.

Case Study 3

1. The evaluation process includes determining dental dam placement, that is, punching holes for the missing/malpositioned teeth, and generally following the patterns of the teeth in the patient's mouth.

2. Holes are often positioned at the buccal or lingual of the arch's normal curve. Corresponding holes must be positioned toward the buccal or the lingual to match the arch.

3. Punching holes for the pontics is not possible; punches are made for the abutment teeth and spaces are left for the number of pontics. Slits are cut between the holes with scissors to allow the bridges to be exposed.

4. The hole is punched facially to its normal position in the arch. A cervical clamp is often used with the Class V restoration, because it retracts the gingiva and the dam beyond the borders of the cavity. The largest hole on the punch is used for this clamp, because the double wings allow an additional 1 to 3 mm between adjacent teeth.

Labeling

See Figure 34–55 in text.

a. vise

b. spindle

c. outer knob

d. guide channels

e. diagonal slot

f. frame

g. inner knob

Laboratory Materials and Techniques

Multiple Choice

1. a	2. b	3. d	4. c	5. b	6. b	7. d
8. b	9. b	10. a	11. d	12. a	13. b	14. c
15. b	16. b	17. b	18. a	19. c	20. c	21. a
22. a	23. a	24. b	25. a	26. b	27. a	28. d
29. a	30. d					

Critical Thinking

1. Both terms—interim restoration and temporaries—are correct. Such restorations must be comfortable and aesthetically acceptable to the patient; remain stable; have proper mesial and distal contacts and occlusal alignment, until the permanent crown is cemented; be easily removed, without damaging the tooth, when the permanent restoration is ready for placement; and fit snugly and accurately along the prepared margin of the tooth. There should be less than 1/2 mm of space between the temporary restoration and the finish line of the margin, and it should be contoured in a similar fashion to the original tooth, protecting the gingiva from irritation and interproximal areas from food impaction.

2. Cut into the crest of the wax making small rectangular or round holes—called stops (holes on the spacer that allow bumps to be formed on the tissue side of the tray). Allow the tray to be seated 2 to 3 mm from the teeth; do not seat too deeply. For crowns or bridges, the stops should be placed one tooth distal and mesial from the prepared tooth. This allows an adequate amount of impression material to flow around the prepared tooth.

3. A frame that holds models of the patient's teeth in order to maintain the patient's occlusal and represent his or her jaws. Used to study malocclusion, carve teeth for crowns and bridges, and demonstrate to the patient the action that is of concern.

4. Both maxillary and mandibular models are trimmed symmetrically following specific cut angles indicated; all the anatomic portion of the model are accurate; the trimmed models sit on end and maintain occlusion; models each exhibit a 1/2-inch base and a 1-inch anatomic portion. The last step is final finishing so that the model presents a professional appearance.

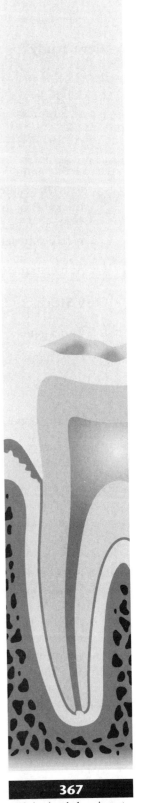

Case Study 1

1. Most offices use preformed aluminum and acrylic crowns, along with custom acrylic or composite crowns.

2. Used by either direct matrix or indirect matrix.

3. Making the matrix directly from the tooth, alginate impression, impression material, or freehand (making a block of the material and covering the prepared tooth).

4. Making the matrix on a model or cast, wax, thermo-forming beads or buttons, or vacuum-formed shell.

Case Study 2

1. The regular stock tray does not fit. The stock tray will not allow a minimum amount of space for the material to flow around the prepared area, or it may require that excessive impression material is used to obtain the impression, therefore risking an inferior outcome.

2. A custom tray can be fabricated to meet the need.

3. Stable enough to hold the material rigid during placement and removal; can be smoothed and contoured to arch; adapted to an edentulous, a partially edentulous, and a full dentition; adapted to allow uniform thickness of impression material in all areas of the arch, and altered and contoured to any irregular area. It can also be designed in such a way that stops are in the spacer, thereby holding the material in a stable, specifically determined area to provide a more accurate impression.

4. Acrylic tray resin self-curing, light-curing, vacuum-formed, and thermoplastic.

Case Study 3

1. Also a generic name used for a group of irreversible hydrocolloid impression materials.

2. Used when less accuracy is needed.

3. Most common areas are used in making diagnostic casts or study models.

4. Making opposing models for fixed and removable prosthetics, orthodontic appliances, mouth guards, bleach trays, provisional restorations, and custom trays.

Dental Office Management

Multiple Choice

1. d	2. b	3. b	4. c	5. b	6. a	7. b
8. c	9. b	10. b	11. b	12. a	13. d	14. b
15. c	16. d	17. a	18. d	19. c	20. a	21. c
22. d	23. c	24. d	25. d			

Matching

Match each term with its description.

1. d   2. c   3. b   4. a

Critical Thinking

1. Answering systems, answering services, voice mail, fax machines, electronic mail (e-mail), cellular phones and services, and paging systems.

2. Protection from computer viruses; firewalls (to limit access to the office intranet to specific computer users) established in the office system; daily backup routines to limit damage resulting from system crashes or spread of computer viruses.

   Computer ergonomics involves implementation of fatigue-reducing and health-sustaining practices (focus on human–tool interface). Examples include keeping wrists in level position, screen glare protectors to deflect and reduce monitor glare, and maintaining aseptic procedures for computer keyboards in treatment rooms and laboratory.

3. Managed care plans provide minimum care for all members, encourage preventive services, and try to control costs (providing high-level care at reduced fees). In capitation programs, medical providers are reimbursed a set fee per patient (as by an HMO) regardless of treatment required.

4. Birthday rule. When both parents have coverage for the child, the rule establishes that the insurance company of the parent whose birthday month and day (not year) comes earlier in the calendar year is the primary carrier.

   Benefit-less-benefit. For patients who are insured by two carriers, reimbursement is limited to the higher level allowed of the two plans.

   Coordination of benefits (COB). When two insurance carriers coordinate the benefits, the total cost of the actual dental treatment expense must not be exceeded.

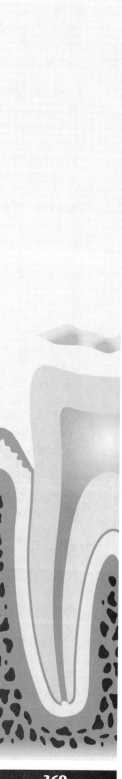

Case Study 1

1. Briefly, such changes can be described as aimed at overcoming the widespread negative image of dentistry. Today, dentistry can be a pain-free and positive experience.

2. Regarding the physical environment, many dentists hire an interior design consultant and/or space-planning advisor to assist in developing spaces that are inviting and pleasant for the patients.

3. Dental receptionist. In the past, the receptionist had a broad range of responsibilities, from greeting patients and scheduling appointments to bookkeeping. Receptionists today must be able to efficiently multitask. Roles may include any one or combination of the following (among others): greeting patients, assisting patients to fill out initial paperwork required for treatment, answering the telephone and taking messages, scheduling appointments, and maintaining patient chart system and records.

   Dental office bookkeeper. Depending on office size, these activities could be shared with the receptionist. All office finances are handled by this person, including accounts receivable and accounts payable. The bookkeeper may also handle patient dental insurance and make financial arrangement for dental service payments, and inventory and supply systems. This person must be organized, be knowledgeable about dental treatments, and exhibit good communication and problem-solving skills.

4. Marketing is a means of attracting new patients and retaining patients. Dental assistants, along with all the members of the dental team, need to be involved in marketing the practice. Methods are quite varied and include, for instance, a monthly newsletter for patients with tips for dental health, and periodic giveaways and flowers distributed to patients at each appointment or sent to patients as referral thank-you's.

Case Study 2

1. File folders, file cabinet, color-coding systems applied to individual files and/or file cabinet holders.

2. The patient chart filing system is organized alphabetically and indexes individual patient names (patient name is divided into last name, first name, and middle name or initial). All charts are filed by patient surname. When duplicate surnames exist, the surname plus first name is used, and if duplicates of these exist, the middle initial is used. Offices may also use color-coding files, tabs, and date stickers. A tickler file serves to remind office staff of future actions.

3. See Chapter 3 for a review of the HIPAA policy. The patient does have a right to confidentiality of treatment and clinical records.

4. Most dentists keep records throughout their entire careers. Record archives may be in hard copy or electronic form (e.g., optical disc), or some combination of these. Electronic archives contain large amounts of data and are easily retrievable (compared to hard copy files).

Case Study 3

1. Under the Fair Debt Collection Practice Act, telephoning a debtor at inconvenient hours is illegal. In addition, collection calls to the debtor's employers, except to verify employment, are prohibited, as are attempting to obtain information under false pretenses or by threatening violence.

2. Verification is necessary to identify the person as the contact individual. Then discuss methods for resolving the problem. Always set a date for when the payment can be expected. If it does not arrive in this time frame, contact the patient immediately to let the patient know that the dental office cannot and will not let the debt "slide."

3. Cash payments, check payments, cashier's checks, credit cards, and loans.

4. If the debtor cannot be reached by telephone, a collection letter is necessary. Collection letters are sent via certified mail. Every effort is made to contact the patient and encourage him or her to pay the overdue balance. Occasionally, the dental office turns highly delinquent accounts over to an outside collection agency. The typical charge for this service is one-third of the balance collected.

CHAPTER 37

Employment Strategies

Multiple Choice

1. c	2. c	3. b	4. d	5. d	6. c	7. d
8. d	9. b	10. c	11. a	12. d	13. b	14. b
15. b	16. c	17. d	18. d	19. d	20. b	21. d
22. c						

Critical Thinking

1. When going to work is simply unpleasant (for whatever reasons), the dental assistant should express his or her concerns with the office manager or dentist. Upon deciding to seek new employment, the assistant should submit a letter of resignation or verbally notify the employer, and allow 2 weeks' notice. Do everything possible to leave a position on good terms with the employer.

2. Always be on time, be ready to perform the necessary skills, plan ahead, and prepare for success. Take care of all outside practical matters, child care, transportation, and backup arrangements as needed. Maintain high standards of personal hygiene and appearance. Know job requirements, and try to go above and beyond these expectations.

3. Now would be the appropriate time to discuss salary. Ask about benefits and learn about office policies, sick days, holidays, and vacation time. Determine all specific dental assistant responsibilities and office hours. Find out when performance evaluations are conducted and what performance objectives lead to a raise in pay.

Case Study 1

1. Dental Assisting National Board, Inc. (DANB).

2. A certificate can be displayed that verifies successful completion of the DANB test. The assistant can also wear the official Certified Dental Assistant (CDA) pin, and use the CDA title.

3. Pathway I as defined by DANB, Pathway II as defined by DANB, and Pathway III as defined by DANB.

4. Plan for the future, continue to improve your dental assisting skills and knowledge base through continuing education, and stay up-to-date on new techniques and materials. Seek out continuing education opportunities through the dental assistant association or other professional groups, as well as local community colleges and 4-year institutions.

5. Ensures that patients receive the best care possible and builds the self-esteem of dental assistants.

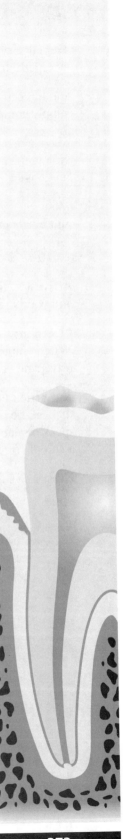

Case Study 2

1. Solo: single dentist.

   Partnership: contractual agreement in which each dentist partner has equal rights and duties.

   Group practice: any number of dentists can share a building and still remain independent.

   Dental specialty practice: examples are oral surgery, endodontics, periodontics, orthodontics, prosthodontics, pathology, pediatric, and dental public health.

2. Public sector dental offices (federal, including veterans hospitals, state, and local), laboratories, dental supply companies, and insurance companies.

3. Make a decision about the type of practice, check the classifieds in daily newspapers, access local dental and dental assistant societies' postings and newsletters, use career placement services in schools, employment agencies, and dental supply companies (staff often know of dentists seeking employees).

4. Many of the sources listed in no. 3 have Web sites. Start with employment searches of dental professions and by geographical location.

Case Study 3

1. Arrive at least 5 minutes early for the interview, do some research on the dental office, and know yourself and your strengths and abilities. Be prepared for the question, "Why should we hire you for this position?"

2. Questions to ask/consider during interview: opportunities and requirements for continuing education. When employment is offered (and not before), questions to ask include specifics on salary, benefits, sick leave, and vacation.

3. Ask a friend or family member to perform a mock interview and provide you with feedback on any areas that can be improved. Practice the following: firm handshake, eye contact, and smile. Sit up straight and speak distinctly. Plan ahead for responses to certain questions and actions, such as what to do when handed a cup of coffee.

4. Dress in a subdued, professional manner for an interview (e.g., no jeans), and demonstrate good hygiene.

Practice Management Software

EXERCISES AND ACTIVITIES

Find the following patients and indicate their date of birth, date of last visit, and if the patient has medical alerts on the line next to each name.

1. Tina Young   11/13/59; 3/21/05; high blood pressure

2. Mark Taylor   7/24/65; 3/14/05; none

3. Rachelle Johnson   4/21/73; 2/1/05; allergies

4. Brent Crosby   5/17/67; 4/14/05; allergy – codeine, allergy – hayfever, dizziness, ulcers

5. Martin Winters   11/29/94; 2/22/05; none

6 through 10 – the student was given patient information to enter on his or her own.

Periodontal Charting

1.

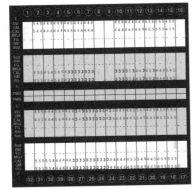

2.

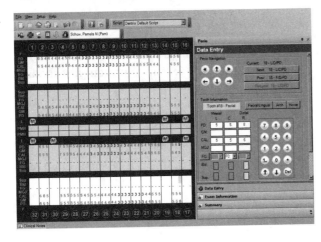

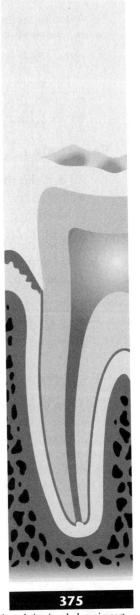

Appointment Scheduling

1 through 5 – the student was given patient information and asked to schedule patients for practice.

Prescriptions

1 through 5 – the student was given patient information and asked to add prescriptions for practice.

Review Patient Management

Multiple Choice

1. a	2. a	3. b	4. a	5. d	6. b	7. b	8. c	9. c
10. d	11. b	12. b	13. c	14. b	15. d	16. a	17. c	18. a

Critical Thinking

1. Benefits of using a computerized appointment book would include automatic tracking of patients, legibility, remote accessibility, and ease of finding/making appointments.

2. Documents are secure because there is no paper containing PHI that could be picked up or seen by dishonest or curious individuals. No paper information needs to leave the office so no charts go off the premises. Data is backed up and stored off premises so in case of a fire or other damage the "charts" stay safe.

3. To keep private information private; place computer screens at an angle they can't be viewed by patients or guests, print only necessary information to eliminate additional paper that must be shredded, and set up secure security systems on your computer system.

Case Study 1

1. All dental staff need to use the computer. It isn't fair to have someone else do Debby's work if she isn't willing to try. Having an employee working in a paperless office without computer skills would reduce productivity.

2. This is where teamwork can be helpful; if Debby is willing to learn, someone should be willing to help her. Long-time employees bring a lot to a practice in terms of knowing the practice and patients and it is worth the time to train them on new technology.

3. Benefits to Debby might be increased production for herself and the team, self-esteem from accomplishing something difficult for her, increased employability, and reduction in stress from constantly looking for charts.

Case Study 2

1. When you open Jim's chart to make his appointment you have immediate access to employer and insurance information, what Jim needs to schedule an appointment for, his past appointment history, any alerts, and appointment information for anyone else on his account.

2. First you would want to confirm any changes in information. Determining changes early can save you from having awkward problems later.

3. By seeing that Jim's family members are also due to make appointments, this can be mentioned or even possibly scheduled while Jim is on the phone.

Practice Management

Multiple Choice

1. b	2. d	3. c	4. a	5. d	6. b	7. d
8. a	9. b	10. b	11. c	12. b	13. c	14. c
15. d	16. a	17. d	18. d	19. a	20. d	

Critical Thinking

1. Everyone in the office should know the basics of creating reports. They assist the staff in achieving goals, and by not having to wait for help running a report the information is available immediately.

2. All correspondence should be read for accuracy. Even preprogrammed letters should be examined. When a bulk mailing is done this is not practical, so entering information accurately is extremely important.

3. Errors continue throughout the system if not corrected. If the charting is incorrect, the patient's clinical chart will contain an error, and all of the billing will be wrong including the ledger and insurance documents.

Case Study 1

1. With practice, tracking down bookkeeping problems is easy. First start with the ledger and examine the timeline of what has occurred. Was the original treatment and posting entered correctly? Was the insurance sent? Has the insurance portion of the account been paid? All of these things can be printed out for the patient so he can easily see his account.

2. If the problem is yours, and it happens, using your reporting systems can be helpful. Tracking unpaid insurance claims can avoid past due accounts and help your practice's cash flow. Staying on top of delinquent accounts is important. Collecting past due accounts is more successful when you monitor them and try to collect before the account is severely delinquent. Dan specifically mentions statements so it appears this has gone on several months—monitoring accounts may have eliminated this scenario.

3. If the problem is because Dan misunderstood how and what his insurance would pay, this can be helpful information. Because informed consent is very important and we need to do the best job possible when presenting cases, DENTRIX® can print out treatment plans that enable patients to have a copy of all the details of treatment proposed and accepted.

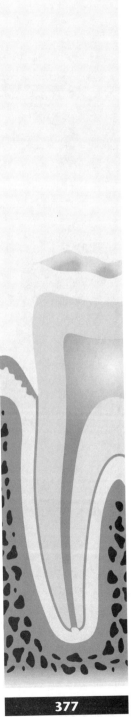

Case Study 2

1. Susan may be accurate and she may not have a separate dental card. Remember you can track her insurance by employer too.

2. After determining the employer, you'd need to know who the primary subscriber is and if any secondary insurance exists. When you have determined those things, you can verify the insurance per your normal office procedure with the information in the software.